NUCLEAR CARDIOLOGY REVIEW

A Self-Assessment Tool

Second Edition

EDITORS

Wael A. Jaber, MD, FACC, FESC

Professor of Medicine
Cleveland Clinic Lerner College of Medicine
Case Western Reserve University
Staff Cardiologist
Heart & Vascular Institute
Cleveland Clinic
Cleveland, Ohio

Manuel D. Cerqueira, MD, FACC, MASNC

Professor of Radiology and Medicine
Cleveland Clinic Lerner College of Medicine
Case Western Reserve University
Chairman
Department of Nuclear Medicine
Imaging Institute
Staff Cardiologist
Heart & Vascular Institute
Cleveland Clinic
Cleveland, Ohio

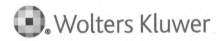

Philadelphia • Baltimore • New York • London
Buenos Aires • Hong Kong • Sydney • Tokyo

Acquisitions Editor: Sharon Zinner
Editorial Coordinator: John Larkin
Marketing Manager: Rachel Mante Leung
Production Project Manager: David Saltzberg
Design Coordinator: Holly Reid McLaughlin
Manufacturing Coordinator: Beth Welsh
Prepress Vendor: SPi Global

Second edition

15 14 13 12 11 10 9

Printed in The United States of America

Library of Congress Cataloging-in-Publication Data
Names: Jaber, Wael A., author, editor. | Cerqueira, Manuel D., author, editor.
Title: Nuclear cardiology review : a self-assessment tool / editors, Wael A. Jaber, Manuel D. Cerqueira.
Description: Second edition. | Philadelphia : Wolters Kluwer, [2018] | Includes bibliographical references and index.
Identifiers: LCCN 2017033411 | ISBN 9781496326928
Subjects: | MESH: Cardiac Imaging Techniques | Cardiovascular Diseases–diagnostic imaging | Heart–diagnostic imaging | Image Interpretation, Computer-Assisted | Radionuclide Imaging–methods | Examination Questions
Classification: LCC RC683.5.R33 | NLM WG 18.2 | DDC 616.1/20754076–dc23 LC record available at https://lccn.loc.gov/2017033411

LWW.com

■

To Lara, Maya, and Roxanne!
WAEL A. JABER, MD, FACC, FESC

■

To Rachel, David, Christina, Gabriella, and Arianna,
who make everything fun and worthwhile.
MANUEL D. CERQUEIRA, MD, FACC, MASNC

CONTRIBUTORS

Kanak Amin, BS
RadioChemist
Department of Nuclear Medicine
Imaging Institute
Cleveland Clinic
Cleveland, Ohio

Richard C. Brunken, MD
Professor of Radiology
Cleveland Clinic Lerner College of Medicine
Case Western Reserve University
Director of Molecular Cardiac Imaging
Department of Nuclear Medicine
Imaging Institute
Cleveland Clinic
Cleveland, Ohio

Manuel D. Cerqueira, MD, FACC, MASNC
Professor of Radiology and Medicine
Cleveland Clinic Lerner College of Medicine
Case Western Reserve University
Chairman
Department of Nuclear Medicine
Imaging Institute
Staff Cardiologist
Heart & Vascular Institute
Cleveland Clinic
Cleveland, Ohio

Paul C. Cremer, MD
Cardiovascular Imaging Associate Staff
Robert & Suzanne Tomsich Department of
Cardiovascular Medicine
Cleveland Clinic
Cleveland, Ohio

Frank P. DiFilippo, PhD, DABSNM
Director of Nuclear Imaging Physics
Department of Nuclear Medicine
Imaging Institute
Cleveland Clinic
Cleveland, Ohio

Wael A. Jaber, MD, FACC, FESC
Professor of Medicine
Cleveland Clinic Lerner College of Medicine
Case Western Reserve University
Staff Cardiologist
Heart & Vascular Institute
Cleveland Clinic
Cleveland, Ohio

Brett W. Sperry, MD
Advanced Heart Failure & Transplant Cardiology
Fellow
Robert & Suzanne Tomsich Department of
Cardiovascular Medicine
Cleveland Clinic
Cleveland, Ohio

Nuclear cardiology has evolved to be the most important and frequently performed cardiovascular imaging modality for stratifying patients at risk for coronary artery disease as well as localizing ischemia in patients with established coronary artery disease pre- and postrevascularization. It was recognized early that with rapid growth and widespread implementation, there is a need to maintain quality by documenting that those physicians involved in performing and interpreting studies have received adequate training and meet and maintain a minimum level of technical and interpretative skills. To that end, the field implemented a voluntary process of physician certification so that practitioners could be evaluated on their knowledge of the basic sciences in nuclear imaging, maintenance of safety and quality, study interpretation, and appropriately applying test results for optimal patient diagnosis and management. Certification was not intended or designed to test for esoteric knowledge but to evaluate the practical technical and clinical skills required to safely and accurately interpret commonly performed nuclear cardiology studies.

Over the past decade, newer applications for nuclear cardiac imaging were introduced including PET imaging for patients with suspected cardiac sarcoidosis, amyloidosis, and even endocarditis. To this end, this update includes almost 100 new questions and refinement of older questions to emphasize newer developments in the field and adherence to appropriate use criteria (AUC).

This updated version of the board review book takes this same practical and pragmatic approach based on our extensive experience in all aspects of nuclear cardiology at the high volume Cleveland Clinic Center. Equal emphasis and importance is given to the technical, interpretative, and clinical application of nuclear cardiology. Aspects of instrumentation, image processing, radiopharmaceuticals, and radiation safety are critical for image interpretation and need to be mastered by those physicians involved in interpreting and using the test results. Test questions are annotated with discussion on image interpretation and technical aspects that may lead to image artifacts.

Wael A. Jaber
Manuel D. Cerqueira

CONTENTS

3D	three-dimensional
AAA	abdominal aortic aneurysm
AC	attenuation correction
ACC	American College of Cardiology
AHA	American Heart Association
ALARA	as low as reasonable achievable
AMI	acute myocardial infarction
ASNC	American Society of Nuclear Cardiology
AV	atrioventricular
BGO	bismuth germanate
BMI	body mass index
CABG	coronary artery bypass graft
CAC	coronary calcium score
CAD	coronary artery disease
CHD	coronary heart disease
CHF	congestive heart failure
COPD	chronic obstructive pulmonary disease
CT	computed tomography
CV	cardiovascular
CZT	cadmium–zinc–telluride
DOT	Department of Transportation
DTPA	diethylamine triamine pentaacetic acid
DTS	Duke Treadmill Score
ECG	electrocardiogram
ED	end diastolic
EF	ejection fraction
EKG	electrocardiogram
ERNA	equilibrium radionuclide angiocardiography
FDA	Food and Drug Administration
FDG	^{18}F-2-fluoro-2-deoxy-2-D-glucose
FDGAC	^{18}F-2-fluoro-2-deoxy-2-D-glucose
FPRNA	first-pass radionuclide angiography
GI	gastrointestinal
GSO	gadolinium oxyorthosilicate
HVL	half value layer
ICD	implantable cardioverter defibrillator
IV	intravenous
LAD	left anterior descending
LBBB	left bundle-branch block
LCX	left circumflex artery
LEHR	low-energy high-resolution

LET	linear transfer energy
LIMA	left internal mammary artery
LSO	lutetium oxyorthosilicate
LV	left ventricular
LVEF	left ventricular ejection fraction
LVH	left ventricular hypertrophy
LYSO	lutetium yttrium orthosilicate
MDCT	multidetector computed tomography
MI	myocardial infarction
MPI	myocardial perfusion imaging
MRI	magnetic resonance imaging
MUGA	multiple gated acquisition
NRC	Nuclear Regulatory Commission
NSR	normal sinus rhythm
NYHA	New York Heart Association
PCI	percutaneous intervention
PET	positron emission tomography
PMT	photo multiplier tube
PND	paroxysmal nocturnal dyspnea
PVC	premature ventricular contraction
QC	quality control
RA	right atrial
RAO	right anterior oblique
RBBB	right bundle-branch block
RBC	red blood cell
RCA	right coronary artery
RNA	radionuclide angiography
RNI	radionuclide imaging
RV	right ventricular
SA	sinoatrial node
SOB	shortness of breath
SPECT	single photon emission computed tomography
SPECT MPI	single photon emission computed tomography myocardial perfusion imaging
STEMI	ST-elevation myocardial infarction
TID	transient ischemic dilation
TIMI	thrombolysis in myocardial infarction
VSD	ventricular septal defect
VT	ventricular tachycardia

Physics and Instrumentation

Kanak Amin, Frank P. DiFilippo, and Wael A. Jaber

QUESTIONS

1. A patient scheduled to undergo chemotherapy for breast carcinoma is referred for baseline equilibrium radionuclide angiocardiography (ERNA) for assessment of left ventricular (LV) function to monitor for cardiotoxicity. Which of the following statements is true?

   A. ERNA utilizes technetium-99m sestamibi to tag red blood cells (RBCs).

   B. Hydralazine, prazosin, heparin, and digoxin improve RBC labeling.

   C. Heart/lung ratio can be calculated with this technique.

   D. When calculating left ventricular ejection fraction (LVEF), background activity is added.

2. Which of the following statements regarding first-pass radionuclide angiography (FPRNA) is true?

   A. FPRNA can detect and quantify left-to-right cardiac shunts.

   B. Technetium-99m diethylaminetriamine pentaacetic acid (DTPA) can be used for FPRNA.

   C. FPRNA can evaluate right and LV systolic function.

   D. Optimal results are achieved in the upright, straight anterior view.

   E. All of the choices.

3. Approximately what fraction of 140 keV gamma rays (technetium-99m) pass through a typical low-energy high-resolution (LEHR) parallel-hole collimator?

    A. 1 in 10 (10%)

    B. 1 in 100 (1%)

    C. 1 in 1,000 (0.1%)

    D. 1 in 10,000 (0.01%)

4. If a gamma camera with parallel-hole collimator is moved farther away from the patient, how are resolution and sensitivity affected?

    A. Resolution worsens, and sensitivity remains approximately constant.

    B. Sensitivity worsens, and resolution remains approximately constant.

    C. Both resolution and sensitivity worsen.

    D. Both resolution and sensitivity remain approximately constant.

5. For thallium-201 imaging, the photons detected in the 70-keV window are produced by which mechanism?

    A. Bremsstrahlung

    B. Gamma-ray emission

    C. Internal conversion

    D. X-ray emission

6. In a planar gated blood pool study, 121,344 net counts are measured in the left ventricle at end diastole, and 53,311 net counts are measured at end systole. What is the LVEF? (Assume that background count subtraction has already been performed.)

    A. 22%

    B. 44%

    C. 56%

    D. 78%

7. Which of the following methods of attenuation correction (AC) is not acceptable for nuclear cardiology?

    A. Transmission source AC

    B. Calculated AC from external boundaries

    C. Computed tomography (CT)-based AC

    D. None of the choices (i.e., all are acceptable)

8. The frequency of energy peaking for a gamma camera should be performed:

    A. Daily.

    B. Weekly.

    C. Only after camera service.

    D. Monthly.

9. The technetium-99m photopeak on a gamma scintillation camera is progressively increasing. The most likely cause for this photopeak shift is:

    A. High-energy collimator.

    B. Energy window set at wrong peak.

    C. High-voltage supply to the photomultiplier tube (PMT).

    D. Software issue.

10. To check if all the PMTs are working properly on a gamma camera, which of the following tests should be performed?

    A. Center of rotation

    B. Linearity

    C. Flood-field uniformity

    D. Resolution

11. The interaction of a technetium-99m gamma photon with the scintillation camera is primarily by:

    A. Compton effect.

    B. Photoelectric effect.

    C. Pair production.

    D. Scatter effect.

12. In order for the technetium-99m peak to be acquired within a 20% window, the window setting should be:

    A. 112 to 168 keV.

    B. 126 to 154 keV.

    C. 0 to 140 keV.

    D. 112 to 140 keV.

13. The best method to check for patient motion on a cardiac single photon emission computed tomography (SPECT) study is to:

    A. Use a ramp filter during reconstruction.

    B. Review the long- and short-axis images.

    C. Check projection images in a cine format.

    D. Ask the technologist if the patient moved.

14. In a cardiac SPECT study, the acquired planar projections are first reconstructed into which body plane?

    A. Transaxial

    B. Long axis

    C. Coronal

    D. Planar

15. In a multigated acquisition (MUGA) study, the cardiac cycle is divided in 20 equal time frames, and the patient heart rate is 60 beats per minute. Average time per frame is:

    A. 5 seconds.

    B. 50 seconds.

    C. 0.05 seconds.

    D. 0.5 seconds.

16. Dual-head camera detectors are mounted next to each other in a 90-degree orientation to the gantry for a cardiac study; this is primarily done because:

    A. The resolution is improved.

    B. The time is reduced in half compared to full 180-degree rotation.

    C. Scatter is reduced.

    D. The resolution is increased.

17. The amount of energy deposited by the radiation per unit length in an absorber is known as:

    A. Specific ionization.

    B. Linear transfer energy (LET).

    C. Range of radiation.

    D. Exposure.

18. Attenuation artifacts are prevalent in SPECT imaging modalities. Which of the following statements is true?

    A. Anterior wall attenuation is present in males more than females.

    B. Specificity of diagnosing right coronary artery (RCA) disease is compromised in male patients.

    C. Gated SPECT images are of little help in ruling out attenuation artifacts.

    D. Attenuation artifacts affect the sensitivity of SPECT imaging but not specificity.

19. Using AC and resolution compensation has been recently introduced in SPECT imaging. This newer technology:

    A. Reduces the sensitivity of SPECT to detect coronary artery disease (CAD).

    B. Improves the sensitivity of SPECT to detect multivessel CAD.

    C. Improves the number of false-negative SPECT studies.

    D. Reduces the number of false-positive SPECT studies.

20. When comparing pharmacologic SPECT versus pharmacologic positron emission tomography (PET), all the following statements are true except:

    A. PET has a higher spatial resolution.

    B. PET perfusion tracers have a shorter half-life.

    C. Quantification of absolute myocardial blood flow is more feasible with PET.

    D. PET agents are readily and widely available.

21. What percentage of 140-keV gamma rays (technetium-99m) is attenuated by 10 cm of water (attenuation coefficient of water at 140 keV = 0.15 cm^{-1})?

    A. 22%

    B. 44%

    C. 56%

    D. 78%

22. In the above situation (technetium-99m in water), the interaction of gamma rays with the medium is dominated by which process?

    A. Photoelectric absorption

    B. Compton scattering

    C. Rayleigh scattering

    D. Pair production

23. Cardiac SPECT cameras currently utilize any of the following collimation methods, except:

    A. Parallel-hole collimation.

    B. Converging collimation.

    C. Diverging collimation.

    D. Pinhole collimation.

24. Some "solid-state" cameras use photodiodes coupled to pixelated scintillation crystals. What is a main advantage of this design, compared to conventional gamma cameras having a large-area scintillation crystal with photomultiplier tubes?

    A. Higher sensitivity

    B. Higher-energy resolution

    C. Higher spatial resolution

    D. Compact size and lower weight

25. Other "solid-state" detectors use semiconductor crystals (such as cadmium–zinc–telluride, CZT) instead of scintillation crystals. What is a main advantage of semiconductor crystals compared to conventional gamma cameras having a large-area scintillation crystal with photomultiplier tubes?

    A. Higher sensitivity

    B. Higher-energy resolution

    C. Higher spatial resolution

    D. Lower cost

26. All of the following are challenges associated with PET/MR for cardiac imaging, *except*:

    A. PET resolution and sensitivity.

    B. Accuracy of PET attenuation correction.

    C. MRI safety associated with cardiac implants.

    D. MRI safety associated with radiopharmaceutical administration.

27. Modern PET scanners can acquire raw data in list mode, as opposed to sinograms. All of the following are advantages of list mode acquisition, except:

    A. Higher count statistics.

    B. Retrospective EKG or respiratory gating.

    C. Troubleshooting patient motion.

    D. Smaller data files (gated and dynamic studies).

28. In the past, SPECT and PET images were reconstructed using the filtered backprojection algorithm. Recently, iterative reconstruction has become common. In advanced implementations of iterative reconstruction, the blur in the raw data associated with the detector and collimator is modeled. This method has all of the following advantages, except:

    A. Better image quality.

    B. Potential for lower radiation dose.

    C. Need to acquire only half the projections.

    D. Ability to recover some spatial resolution.

29. When using iterative reconstruction, the number of iterations is specified for stopping the program. Why is this done?

    A. To prevent impractical computation time

    B. To control excessive image noise

    C. To optimize the spatial resolution

    D. To match the number of projections (equal to iterations x subsets)

30. For cardiac PET acquired with a PET/CT, why is it important to control the respiratory phase of the CT portion of the examination?

    A. The respiratory phase affects the myocardial distribution of FDG.

    B. The respiratory phase affects the myocardial distribution of the perfusion tracer (ammonia or rubidium).

    C. The respiratory phase affects PET attenuation correction.

    D. The respiratory phase affects scatter in the PET data.

31. Which method of cardiac PET attenuation correction is not susceptible to artifact from metallic implants?

    A. Transmission attenuation correction (using external ^{68}Ge or ^{137}Cs sources).

    B. CT-based attenuation correction.

    C. MR-based attenuation correction.

    D. All are not affected by metallic implants.

32. A cardiac imaging department (without access to ^{13}N-ammonia or a ^{82}Rb generator) wishes to perform a rest/stress ^{99m}Tc SPECT study in addition to a viability ^{18}F-FDG PET study, on the same day. In which order should these studies be scheduled?

    A. First perform the ^{18}F-FDG PET study and then followed by the rest/stress ^{99m}Tc SPECT study.

    B. First perform the rest/stress ^{99m}Tc SPECT study and then followed by the ^{18}F-FDG PET study.

    C. Perform the ^{18}F-FDG PET study in between the rest and stress ^{99m}Tc SPECT study.

    D. The order does not matter. Any of the above is acceptable.

ANSWERS

1. ANSWER: C. Technetium-99m is used to radiolabel the patient's RBCs. There are three methods for radiolabeling: in vivo, in vitro, and in vivitro. For in vivo labeling, the patient receives intravenous stannous pyrophosphate 15 minutes prior to injection of 15 to 30 millicuries of technetium-99m pertechnetate. This method is the fastest and least expensive but has the lowest labeling efficiency of the RBCs and has a high background due to non-specific labeling of circulating proteins. For the in vitro method, 10 to 15 mL of the patient's blood is drawn, and the stannous pyrophosphate and technetium-99m are added outside the body. Once labeling has been completed, the RBCs are reinjected into the patient. A commercial kit called Ultratag is available. This technique results in the highest labeling efficiency and lowest background activity but is more expensive and time consuming. The third method involves intravenous injection of the stannous pyrophosphate prior to removal of 10 to 15 mL of the patient's RBCs that are then mixed with the technetium-99m pertechnetate.

There are many frequently used medications (hydralazine, prazosin, heparin, and digoxin) that inhibit binding of the technetium-99m pertechnetate to the hemoglobin molecule inside the RBCs. Poor binding is easily detected by finding free technetium-99m pertechnetate in the mucosa of the stomach and in the thyroid gland.

LVEF is calculated by measuring LV counts at end systole and end diastole and correcting for background activity due to overlying radioactivity and background scatter adjacent to the lateral or inferoapical walls of the ventricle. Failure to correct for background activity results in a lower ejection fraction measurement.

LVEF = Background corrected end diastolic counts–Background corrected end systolic counts/Background corrected end diastolic counts.

Heart/lung ratio can be calculated by this technique. This ratio measures how well the ventricles compensate by comparing the counts in the heart and lung. Pooling of blood in the lungs has been reported to be present in heart failure.

The assessment of left ventricle and right ventricle (RV) using ERNA is a class I indication in the ACC/AHA Radionuclide Guidelines. The majority of other indications fall in the class II and III categories.

REFERENCE:

Corbett JR, Akinboboye OO, Bacharach SL, et al.; Quality Assurance Committee of the American Society of Nuclear Cardiology. Equilibrium radionuclide angiocardiography. *J Nucl Cardiol.* 2006;13(6):e56–e79.

2. ANSWER: E. In addition to measuring LV and RV function, FPRNA can also detect and quantify atrial and ventricular shunts. DTPA, cleared by the kidneys, and technetium-99m sulfur colloid, cleared by the liver, give accurate results. Technetium-99m sestamibi and tetrofosmin used to assess myocardial perfusion at rest or peak stress can be given as a bolus for FPRNA when concentrated in a sufficiently small volume, ideally 0.5 to 1 mL. FPRNA can be performed when doing an ERNA study by the in vivo method but not when labeling is performed by in vitro or in vivitro methods due to the large volume administered. For timing purposes and quality of image (count density), large veins close to the heart are required for the rapid bolus of DTPA. The straight upright anterior view has the advantage of stabilizing the patient's chest against the detector and positioning the patient so that the right and left ventricles will be in the field of view. FPRNA allows for RV function assessment. A shallow right anterior oblique (RAO) view is recommended to enhance right atrial–RV separation.

REFERENCE:

Friedman JD, Berman DS, Borges-Neto S, et al.; Quality Assurance Committee of the American Society of Nuclear Cardiology. First-pass radionuclide angiography. *J Nucl Cardiol.* 2006;13(6):e42–e55.

3. ANSWER: D. A typical LEHR collimator has a sensitivity of around 200 cpm/μCi for technetium-99m, which equals $(3.3 \text{ cps})/(3.7 \times 10^4 \text{ Bq}) = 0.9 \times 10^{-4}$ cps/Bq. Considering that the crystal efficiency is about 90% and that the 140-keV emission efficiency of technetium-99m is 89%, the collimator efficiency is 1.1×10^{-4}, or about 1 in 10,000.

4. ANSWER: A. Collimator blur increases with distance, and thus, resolution worsens. The number of counts passing through the collimator does not change appreciably as distance increases.

5. ANSWER: D. Thallium-201 decays by electron capture to mercury-201. The mercury-201 is in an excited state and releases x-rays with energies near 70 keV.

6. ANSWER: C. The difference between the net counts ($121,344 - 53,311 = 68,033$) indicates the activity ejected by the left ventricle. The ejection fraction is ($68,033/121,344$) = 56%.

7. ANSWER: B. Transmission and CT-based AC use a radioactive source or CT to create density or attenuation maps that are applied to the emission activity from the heart during reconstruction. Calculated AC does not directly measure the attenuation but calculates it based on assumptions of uniform attenuation and has been used successfully for brain SPECT or PET since the attenuation coefficient is approximately constant over the entire slice. However, for cardiac imaging, there is large variance in attenuation coefficient (lungs vs. other tissues such as diaphragm and breast), and calculated methods are not reliable.

8. ANSWER: A. The gamma camera should be checked each day before use to ensure that the energy window has not drifted and the energy spectrum is of the appropriated shape. The energy spectrum of a radionuclide source is acquired, and the photopeak is checked (either automatically or visually) to confirm that it is centered in the energy window.

REFERENCES:

Early PJ, Sodee DB. *Principles and Practice of Nuclear Medicine.* 2nd ed. St. Louis, MO: Mosby; 1985.
Saha GB. *Fundamentals of Nuclear Medicine.* 5th ed. New York, NY: Springer-Verlag; 1993.
Saha GB. *Physics and Radiobiology of Nuclear Medicine.* 3rd ed. New York, NY: Springer-Verlag; 1993.

9. ANSWER: C. The PMT consists of a photocathode that is light sensitive and a series of metallic plates (dynodes). A high voltage is applied to the plates, and when a light photon strikes the crystal, the photoelectron is absorbed by the photocathode and is multiplied by each dynode and a pulse is generated, which is proportional to the amount of energy of the isotope interacting with the crystal. The voltage to these plates has to be very stable, and a slight variation will greatly affect the pulse generated.

REFERENCES:

Early PJ, Sodee DB. *Principles and Practice of Nuclear Medicine*. 2nd ed. St. Louis, MO: Mosby; 1995.
Saha GB. *Physics and Radiobiology of Nuclear Medicine*. 3rd ed. New York, NY: Springer-Verlag; 1993.

10. ANSWER: C. A uniform source of radioactive source (flood sheet) is placed on the camera detector to check if all the PMTs are operational. If a PMT tube is malfunctioning, then a blank spot is observed on the flood scan. The large white area in the lower right corner shows the abnormality (Fig. 1.1). The rest of the detector is uniform.

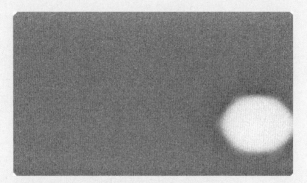

Figure 1.1

REFERENCES:

Early PJ, Sodee DB. *Principles and Practice of Nuclear Medicine*. 2nd ed. St. Louis, MO: Mosby; 1995.
Saha GB. *Fundamentals of Nuclear Medicine*. 5th ed. New York, NY: Springer-Verlag; 1993.
Saha GB. *Physics and Radiobiology of Nuclear Medicine*. 3rd ed. New York, NY: Springer-Verlag; 1993.

11. ANSWER: B. In photoelectric absorption, the gamma ray transfers all its energy to an orbital electron of the absorbing material and a photoelectron is released. Compton scatter occurs when the gamma photon transfers only part of its energy to an orbital electron. The scattered photon travels in a different direction and may further interact in the material.

REFERENCES:

Early PJ, Sodee DB. *Principles and Practice of Nuclear Medicine*. 2nd ed. St. Louis, MO: Mosby; 1995.
Saha GB. *Physics and Radiobiology of Nuclear Medicine*. 3rd ed. New York, NY: Springer-Verlag; 1993.

12. ANSWER: B. Technetium-99m has a mean photopeak energy of 140 keV. In order to set a 20% window centered on the photopeak, the window width is 140 × 0.2 = 28. This gives a range of 14 keV on either side of 140 keV; thus, the energy window limits are 126 to 154 keV.

REFERENCE:

Saha GB. *Physics and Radiobiology of Nuclear medicine.* 3rd ed. New York, NY: Springer-Verlag; 1993.

13. ANSWER: C. A ramp filter is routinely used during reconstruction by filtered backprojection and does not give any information on motion.

Motion during acquisition may give the following artifacts: misalignment of the apex, matching 180-degree areas of decreased intensity in the anterior and inferior walls, hotspots in the septum or lateral wall, and "blobs" or a ring of activity in the anterior wall or an apical nipple. However, seeing such artifacts on the long- and short-axis images does not confirm that there was motion. Review of the raw projection images in a cine format allows visual detection of vertical or up-and-down motion. This can be corrected using motion correction or, if it is excessive, reacquiring the study. Horizontal or side-to-side motion is difficult to detect and cannot be corrected. Rapid or deep breathing may also cause motion like artifacts. Acquisition with a dual-head camera will sometimes give the appearance of motion as the images from each head are displayed in a continuous loop. The last acquisition from one head is displayed next to the first acquisition from the other head. Spatially, these images are adjacent, but temporally, one is at the end and the other at the beginning of acquisition. If the patient moved gradually, such motion may not be detected on individual projections but is seen in the transition from one head to the other. Such motion should not be motion corrected.

The technologist should be questioned, but this in itself is not sufficient as he or she may not have been observing the patient throughout the study.

REFERENCE:

Christian PE, Waterstram-Rich K. *Nuclear Medicine and PET/CT: Technology and Techniques.* 6th ed. St. Louis, MO: Mosby/Elsevier; 2007.

14. ANSWER: A. Thirty-two to sixty-four planar projections are acquired 180 degrees around the patient perpendicular to the long axis of the body, and the initial reconstruction is into the transaxial plane. From these trans-axial images, the long axis of the heart is defined, and subsequently, the conventional vertical and horizontal long-axis and the short-axis images are reconstructed for analysis.

REFERENCE:

Christian PE. *Nuclear Medicine and PET Technology and Techniques.* St. Louis, MO: Mosby; 1981.

15. ANSWER: C.
60 s/(heart rate × the number of frames)
60/(60 × 20) = 0.05

REFERENCE:

Christian PE. *Nuclear Medicine and PET Technology and Techniques.* St. Louis, MO: Mosby; 1981.

16. ANSWER: B. In a cardiac SPECT study, typically 64 projections are obtained over 180 degrees at 3-degree increments, and each projection usually takes about 20 seconds. A total of ~21 minutes will be required. However, if two detectors at 90-degree orientation are used, the time to acquire the 64 projection will be half (11 minutes).

REFERENCE:

Christian PE. *Nuclear Medicine and PET Technology and Techniques*. St. Louis, MO: Mosby; 1981.

17. ANSWER: B. LET is the amount of energy deposited per unit length of the absorber, and units are expressed as keV/μm. Electromagnetic and beta particles have low LET, since they lose little energy per interaction. Alpha particles are heavy particles and lose energy very rapidly and have high LET.

REFERENCE:

Early PJ, Sodee DB. *Principles and Practice of Nuclear Medicine*. 2nd ed. St. Louis, MO: Mosby; 1995.

18. ANSWER: B. Inferior wall attenuation is often present in male patients (diaphragmatic attenuation), and anterior attenuation is often seen in female patients (breast attenuation). These artifacts often affect the specificity of diagnosing CAD by introducing false-positive tests. Normal systolic thickening on gated SPECT in a fixed defect on both rest and stress images represents an attenuation artifact rather than a myocardial scar, which is associated with reduced systolic thickening.

19. ANSWER: D. AC significantly improved the normalcy rate compared to uncorrected perfusion data using either the corrected images (96% vs. 86%) or the corrected data and quantitative analysis (97% vs. 86%). There is no impact on overall sensitivity (75% to 78%), although the detection of multivessel disease was reduced.

REFERENCES:

Hendel RC, Berman DS, Cullom J, et al. Multicenter clinical trial to evaluate the efficacy of correction for photon attenuation and scatter in SPECT myocardial perfusion imaging. *Circulation*. 1999;99:2742.

Hendel RC, Corbett JR, Cullom SJ, et al. The value and practice of attenuation correction for myocardial perfusion SPECT imaging: a joint position statement from the American Society of Nuclear Cardiology and the Society of Nuclear Medicine. *J Nucl Cardiol*. 2002;9:135.

20. ANSWER: D. PET agents used currently for perfusion (rubidium-82 and ^{13}N-ammonia) have limited availability.

21. ANSWER: D. The fraction of nonattenuated gamma rays is given by $e^{-\mu x} = 0.22$, where μ is the attenuation coefficient and x is the length. The percent attenuated is $(1 - 0.22) \times 100\% = 78\%$.

22. ANSWER: B. Compton scattering dominates. Photoelectric absorption is approximately proportional to Z^3/E^3 and is negligible at 140 keV for a low-Z material like water. Rayleigh scattering is not significant at photon energies used in nuclear medicine. Pair production requires photon energies of at least 1.02 MeV (=2 × 511 keV).

23. ANSWER: C. Nearly all SPECT cameras use parallel-hole collimation. Some new designs use converging collimation, such as fan-beam, cone-beam, or cardiofocal collimation. The advantage of converging collimator is that the heart is projected over a large area of the detector, providing higher sensitivity than parallel-hole collimation. Another new design uses multipinhole collimation, where several miniature detectors each having a pinhole collimator are arranged so that the pinholes are all focused on the heart. Higher sensitivity and higher resolution are possible with a multipinhole design. Diverging collimation is really no longer used. In the early years of nuclear medicine, when only detectors with small field of view were available, diverging collimators were used to image a larger field of view with such small detectors.

24. ANSWER: D. Photomultiplier tubes (PMTs) are several inches long. As a result, a gamma camera is about a foot or more in depth and is very heavy, since it is surrounded by thick lead shielding. Solid-state photodiodes are very thin. Detectors using this technology are very compact and lightweight and thus can be used in small cameras suitable for cardiac imaging. Sensitivity is governed mainly by the collimator design, assuming that the crystal has sufficient thickness to absorb most emission photons. Energy resolution of this type of solid-state detector is comparable to or a bit worse than a conventional gamma camera. Spatial resolution depends mainly on the collimator design and to a lesser extent by the detector's intrinsic resolution. Resolution is comparable to a conventional gamma camera.

25. ANSWER: B. In a semiconductor solid-state detector, the electrons produced by absorption of an emission photon are amplified and detected directly. This is much more efficient compared to a scintillation detector, which involves several steps: conversion of electrons to scintillation photons, transport of scintillation photons to the photomultiplier tubes (PMTs), conversion of scintillation photons into electrons in the photocathodes of the PMTs, and amplification and detection of electrons in the PMTs. As a result, the detected electrons in the solid-state detector have better statistical accuracy, and the energy resolution is higher. Sensitivity is governed mainly by the collimator design, assuming that the crystal has sufficient thickness to absorb most emission photons. Although the intrinsic spatial resolution of a semiconductor solid-state detector is often better than that of a conventional gamma camera, the extrinsic spatial resolution depends mainly on the collimator design. Unfortunately, the cost per unit area of semiconductor solid-state detectors is much higher than that of a conventional gamma camera. Thus, solid-state detectors are only practical with clever camera designs using small-area detectors, such as multipinhole collimation or multiple pivoting small detectors.

26. ANSWER: A. PET resolution and sensitivity for PET/MR are comparable to PET/CT. Other factors of PET performance, such as time-of-flight capability and maximum count rate, vary between different PET/CT and PET/MR scanner designs, although both types of scanners produce excellent PET image quality. However, PET attenuation correction based on MRI images has limited accuracy. Unlike CT images, MRI images do not reflect photon attenuation; for example, bone may appear similar to air in an MRI image, but its photon attenuation is higher than soft tissue. Metallic implants typically cause large photopenic regions in MRI images and would cause significant errors in PET attenuation correction. Cardiac implants often are not MRI compatible, and patients must be screened prior to an MRI examination. MRI-compatible rubidium-82 infusion carts currently are not available. If other PET radiopharmaceuticals (FDG, ammonia) are to be administered in the PET/MR room, then only MRI-compatible dose shields, containers, and syringe shields can be used.

27. ANSWER: A. In list mode acquisition, the location and timing of each event is stored in a list. Gated and dynamic studies often can be stored more efficiently in list mode, resulting in smaller data files. The ability to rehistogram the data from a list file allows much greater flexibility in processing data versus sinogram-based acquisition. Studies can be retrospectively processed with different gating parameters or different timing of dynamic sequences. Since PET is a fully 3D acquisition, there are no rotating raw data projections as in SPECT for evaluating patient motion. However, list mode acquisition offers the ability to retrospectively reconstruct various time intervals of the data, for evaluating when motion occurred and for reconstructing images over a time interval determined to have minimal motion. Although list mode acquisition offers great flexibility in data processing, it does not change the sensitivity of the camera or increase the number of counts acquired.

28. ANSWER: C. By modeling the scanner's inherent resolution (also known as the point spread function), the spatial resolution is enhanced to some degree. With equal scan time and injected dose, image quality has been shown to improve when using the more accurate model of the system. Alternatively, similar image quality may be attained with fewer counts, which is a feature sometimes advertised as "half-time imaging." One approach is to reduce injected activity and thereby reduce radiation dose to the patient. Another approach is to reduce scan time and thereby improve throughput and minimize patient motion, which should improve image quality. In this case, the same number of SPECT projections would be acquired, but the time per projection would be reduced.

29. ANSWER: B. A sufficient number of iterations is necessary to ensure convergence and accuracy. However, a large number of iterations amplifies noise. A typical clinical protocol specifies an optimal number of iterations to limit noise while ensuring accuracy, along with a filter to smooth out fluctuations in the reconstructed images. With modern computers, computation time for iterative reconstruction is quite practical. Fast computation is enhanced by processing a subset of the raw data at each iteration, which accelerates convergence. The number of projections is divisible by the number of subsets. However, the total number of iterative updates does not depend on the number of projections; instead, the number of iterations is chosen to prevent noise amplification. Once acceptable convergence is reached, the number of iterations does not affect spatial resolution.

30. ANSWER: C. Traditional dedicated PET scanners (non-CT) acquire transmission attenuation data under free-breathing conditions, so the anatomy of the attenuation map matches that of the PET data, which is also acquired under free-breathing conditions. However with PET/CT, the CT images are acquired very rapidly, and the anatomy of the CT images corresponds to a specific respiratory phase as the beam passes each slice and may not match the anatomy of the PET data. Under free breathing (PET), most of the data are acquired near end expiration. If the lungs are inflated in the CT images, the position of the heart shifts relative to the PET data. For example, the lateral wall of the myocardium in the CT images corresponds to the lung region of the PET data. As a result, CT-based attenuation correction (CT-AC) underestimates the attenuation of the PET lateral wall and could cause a significant artefactual defect. Thus, it is important during CT-AC acquisition to ensure that the respiratory phase is near end expiration to best match the anatomy of the free-breathing PET scan.

REFERENCE:

Gould KL, Pan T, Loghin C, et al. Frequent diagnostic errors in cardiac PET/CT due to misregistration of CT attenuation and emission PET images: a definitive analysis of causes, consequences, and corrections. *J Nucl Med.* 2007;48:1112–1121.

31. ANSWER: A. PET photons have high energy (511 keV) and interact with all materials predominantly by Compton scattering. Transmission imaging with external sources involves photons with the same or similar energy, and the measurement of attenuation is accurate for PET attenuation correction for both body tissue and metallic implants. CT photons, on the other hand, have much lower energy (mostly in the 40 to 100 keV range). These lower energy photons interact with soft tissue primarily by Compton scattering; however, they interact with metallic implants primarily by photoelectric absorption and are much more strongly absorbed. Thus, the CT image significantly overestimates the attenuation of metallic implants. When the CT image is used for PET attenuation correction, it overcorrects for attenuation and could result in artificially high uptake near the implant. Some implants are contraindicated with MR scanning and must be screened prior to imaging. Metallic implants can produce large photopenic regions in MR images, which would severely undercorrect for attenuation if used for PET attenuation correction.

REFERENCE:

DiFilippo FP, Brunken RC. Do implanted pacemaker leads and ICD leads cause metal-related artifact in cardiac PET/CT? *J Nucl Med.* 2005;46:436–443.

32. ANSWER: B. SPECT collimators for ^{99m}Tc imaging are designated as "low-energy collimators" and are designed to collimate 140 keV photons. High-energy photons from ^{18}F easily penetrate through the collimator and would contribute excessive background counts in the ^{99m}Tc SPECT images. A PET scanner operates in coincidence mode, only counting events when two 511 keV photons are detected simultaneously. Single photons from ^{99m}Tc decay are not counted. Thus, it is acceptable to have both ^{18}F and ^{99m}Tc in the patient during a PET scan, but not during a SPECT scan. One cautionary note is that certain PET detectors of older design may exhibit high dead time when high doses of ^{18}F and ^{99m}Tc are in the field of view, in which case it would be beneficial to wait a couple hours after the SPECT scan before performing the PET scan. However, this is not a problem with new PET detector technology.

Radiopharmaceuticals and Radiation Safety

CHAPTER 2

Kanak Amin, Frank P. DiFilippo, and Wael A. Jaber

QUESTIONS

1. Rank the following radionuclides in order of their half-lives (from shortest to longest):

    A. Technetium-99m, fluorine-18, cobalt-57, thallium-201

    B. Fluorine-18, technetium-99m, thallium-201, cobalt-57

    C. Fluorine-18, cobalt-57, technetium-99m, thallium-201

    D. Technetium-99m, fluorine-18, thallium-201, cobalt-57

2. If a radiopharmaceutical labeled with technetium-99m (physical half-life T_p = 6 hours) has a biologic half-life (T_b) of 3 hours, then what is the effective half-life (T_e)?

    A. 1 hour

    B. 2 hours

    C. 3 hours

    D. Cannot be determined from the given information

3. Which of the following radionuclides is useful for quality assurance and calibration of positron emission tomography (PET) scanners?

    A. Germanium-68

    B. Technetium-99m

    C. Cobalt-57

    D. Iodine-131

4. For a same-day myocardial perfusion study using thallium-201-chloride and technetium-99m-sestamibi, which radiopharmaceutical should be scanned first and why?

   A. Technetium-99m-sestamibi should be first, because of its shorter half-life.

   B. Technetium-99m-sestamibi should be first, to maximize image counts.

   C. Thallium-201-chloride should be first, to minimize scatter contamination.

   D. Thallium-201-chloride should be first, to minimize radiation dose to the patient.

5. Which PET radionuclide is produced from a generator?

   A. Carbon-11

   B. Nitrogen-13

   C. Fluorine-18

   D. Rubidium-82

6. A 65-year-old male presents with atrial fibrillation. He was started on a heparin drip. A multigated (MUGA) acquisition scan was ordered to evaluate the left ventricular ejection fraction (LVEF); the most appropriate choice for labeling the red blood cell (RBC) for this patient would be:

   A. Sn-Pyrophate.

   B. Ultratag.

   C. Technetium-99m-tetrofosmin.

   D. Technetium-99m-sestamibi.

7. Technetium-99m has a half-value layer (HVL) of 0.3 mm for lead. How many HVLs are needed to reduce the exposure from a 5-mR exposure to 0.7 mR?

   A. 2 HVLs

   B. 3 HVLs

   C. 1 HVLs

   D. 1.5 HVLs

8. Which of the following is not required under the Nuclear Regulatory Commission (NRC) regulations for the possession of radioactive material?

    A. Limits of radioactive material possessed at any given time

    B. Disposal of radioactive material

    C. Use of radioactive material

    D. Cost of the radioactive material

9. In an unrestricted area of a nuclear imaging facility, which of the following signs is posted?

    A. Caution: Radioactive Material

    B. Caution: Radioactive Area

    C. Danger: Radiation Area

    D. None of the above (no posting required)

10. Caution: Very High Radiation Area sign should be posted in an area where radiation exceeds:

    A. 100 rads per hour.

    B. 200 rads per hour.

    C. 0.2 mrem per hour.

    D. 500 rads per hour.

11. Which of the following areas is considered a restricted area?

    A. Hallways

    B. Where radioactive material is stored and used (hot lab)

    C. Reading room

    D. Scanning room

12. Transportation index found on radioactive shipment packages is a measurement of:

    A. Box type used.

    B. Amount of radioactive material in the package.

    C. Exposure measurement at 1 m from the surface of the package.

    D. Exposure measurement at the surface of the packages.

13. Which of the following instruments is used to measure removable contamination on a radioactive package?

    A. Dose calibrator

    B. Ionization chamber

    C. Well counter

    D. Geiger counter

14. A patient, who is breast-feeding, is scheduled for an exercise stress thallium-201 study. What instruction is critical to be given to the patient before the test is performed?

    A. Abstain from caffeine for 24 hours.

    B. Discontinue all antianginal medications for 24 hours.

    C. Discontinue breast-feeding for 2 weeks after the test.

    D. No instructions needed.

15. Which of the following monitoring devices is most appropriate for the measurement of occupational dose for a radiation worker?

    A. Photographic film badges

    B. Thermoluminescent ring badge

    C. Survey meter

    D. Geiger counter

16. The NRC annual body radiation exposure limit for a radiation is:

    A. 1.25 rem per quarter year.

    B. 50 rem per quarter year.

    C. 15 rem per quarter year.

    D. 50 rem per year.

17. Which of the following radioactive materials can be released into the sewer system?

    A. Unused radioactive patient doses

    B. Sealed radioactive sources

    C. Patient urine or feces

    D. Contaminated paper towel used to clean spill

18. What survey frequency is mandated by the NRC for radioactive materials areas?

    A. Daily

    B. Weekly

    C. Monthly

    D. Yearly

19. Radioactive contamination on the skin is best removed by:

    A. Cleaning with paper towels.

    B. Cleaning with stiff brush.

    C. Cleaning with hot water and soap.

    D. Cleaning with lukewarm water and soap.

20. The maximum exposure amount allowed by the NRC to a fetus of a pregnant occupational worker is:

    A. 500 mrem per month of pregnancy.

    B. 500 mrem per quarter of pregnancy.

    C. 500 mrem for the entire pregnancy.

    D. 50 mrem for the entire pregnancy.

21. The amount of radiation exposure can be reduced by:

    A. Time.

    B. Distance.

    C. Shielding.

    D. All of the choices.

22. A patient undergoing a cardiac stress test is administered technetium-99m-sestamibi. The effective half-life for the heart is 3 hours. What is the biologic half-life?

    A. 3 hours

    B. 6 hours

    C. 2 hours

    D. 1.5 hours

23. A package containing radioactive material is received in the hot lab and found to have a radiation exposure of 5 mR/h at the surface and 0.2 mR/h at 1 m from the surface. Under which of the following Department of Transportation (DOT) labeling categories was the package shipped?

    A. White I

    B. Yellow II

    C. Yellow III

    D. Limited Quantity Shipment

24. For laboratory efficiency and patient convenience, most technetium-99m protocols are performed in 1 day using a rest/stress sequence. How long after the resting injection should the acquisition be performed?

    A. Immediately

    B. 15 minutes

    C. 30 minutes

    D. 2 hours

25. A patient undergoes a 1-day rest/stress technetium-99m single photon emission computed tomography (SPECT) myocardial perfusion study. What is the dose range for the resting study?

    A. 8 to 12 mCi

    B. 15 to 20 mCi

    C. 24 to 36 mCi

    D. 45 mCi

26. Technetium-99m–labeled perfusion tracers have improved SPECT perfusion imaging relative to thallium-201 due to which characteristic?

    A. Longer half-life allowing administration of a higher dose

    B. Higher photon energy resulting in less tissue attenuation

    C. Higher liver and gastrointestinal (GI) uptake

    D. Higher extraction fraction across the coronary bed

27. Attenuation correction techniques have which of the following in common?

   A. A patient-specific attenuation map is created.

   B. All techniques are generated by an x-ray of the patient.

   C. A standard method of attenuation correction has been applied industry wide.

   D. Attenuation correction increases the percent of studies that are read as abnormal.

28. Quantitative analysis and attenuation correction have both been used to improve the diagnostic accuracy of SPECT myocardial perfusion imaging. The interaction between these two methods is best described in which statement?

   A. In contrast to uncorrected SPECT studies, there is no difference in perfusion distributions between normal men and women with attenuation-corrected studies.

   B. More studies are interpreted as normal with quantitative analysis than with attenuation correction.

   C. The specificity of attenuation-corrected images is lower than the images interpreted with quantitative analysis.

   D. Both of these methods lead to a lower sensitivity to detect coronary artery disease.

29. The maximum permissible activity concentration of molybdenum-99 to technetium 99m as stipulated by NRC is:

   A. 0.15 μCi/mCi at the time of elution of technetium-99m from the generator.

   B. 0.15 μCi/mCi at expiration time of technetium-99m.

   C. 0.15 μCi/mCi at the time of administration to the patient.

   D. 0.15 μCi/mCi at the time of compounding with radiopharmaceuticals.

30. Aluminum ion concentration in technetium-99 is regulated by NRC.

   A. True

   B. False

31. When a radioactivity package is delivered to the hot lab of a nuclear medicine department, when must the package be monitored for radioactive contamination?

    A. Within 3 hours after receiving in the hot lab.

    B. Within 3 hours after receiving in the hot lab or within 3 hours from the beginning of the next working day, if received after working hours.

    C. Within 1 hour after receiving in the hot lab.

    D. Radioactive packages must be monitored immediately after receipt.

32. Members of the public in the United States are subject to ionization radiation exposure from natural and man-made radiation sources. On average, they receive approximately half from natural occurring and the other half from man-made, predominantly medical, sources. How much is received annually from all sources?

    A. 620 millirem (6.2 mSv) per year

    B. 310 millirem (3.1 mSv) per year

    C. 620 millirem (6.2 mSv) per adult

    D. 310 millirem (3.1 mSv) per adult

33. How should technenium-99m radioactive waste generated in a nuclear medicine department be disposed?

    A. Store in lead box indefinitely.

    B. Dispose to landfill.

    C. Store in-house for decay to background radiation level before disposal.

    D. Send to approved NRC site for disposal.

ANSWERS

1. ANSWER: B. The half-lives of fluorine-18, technetium-99m, thallium-201, and cobalt-57 are 110 minutes, 6.0 hours, 3.04 days, and 271.7 days, respectively.

2. ANSWER: B. The relationship is given by $(1/T_e) = (1/T_p) + (1/T_b)$.

3. ANSWER: A. Germanium-68 is long-lived (half-life = 271 days) and decays to the positron-emitting gallium-68 (half-life = 68 minutes), so a sealed germanium-68/gallium-68 source behaves in effect like a long-lived positron emitter. The other three choices emit single photons and are useless for PET scanners.

4. ANSWER: C. A main concern for image quality is that a large number of scattered technetium-99m gamma rays are detected in the 70-keV window of thallium-201, and thus, thallium-201 should be imaged first. The technetium-99m half-life is 6 hours, so technetium-99m persists for a same-day study and produces sufficient counts. The order of the studies does not reduce radiation dose.

5. ANSWER: D. Rubidium-82 is the daughter of strontium-82 (half-life = 25 days) and is eluted from a strontium-82/rubidium-82 generator. The other three choices are produced in medical cyclotrons.

6. ANSWER: B. Ultratag is supplied commercially by Mallinckrodt Medical and has stannous citrate along with acid citrate dextrose and sodium hypochlorite. Labeling RBCs using this pharmaceutical is by in vitro method. One to three milliliters of heparinized blood is added to the vial containing stannous citrate and incubated at room temperature for 5 minutes. During the incubation period, the stannous ion diffuses the RBC membrane after which sodium hypochlorite along with acid citrate dextrose is added to the reaction vial, followed by the addition of 30 to 40 millicuries of sodium pertechnetate-technetium-99m and incubation for another 20 minutes. With the addition of implantable cardioverter defibrillator (ICD), the extracellular stannous ion is oxidized by the sodium hypochlorite. The pertechnetate-technetium-99m diffuses the RBC membrane and is reduced intercellularly by the stannous ions. Reduced pertechnetate-technetium-99m does not diffuse out of the RBC. Typical labeling efficiency is >97%.

Heparin is one of the drugs that inhibit the diffusion of stannous ion to the RBC with the use of Sn-Pyrophate, and the labeling is compromised in that some of technetium-99m-pertechnetate is reduced.

REFERENCES:

Package Insert. Ultratag RBC kit for the preparation of Technetium-Tc99m labeled Red Blood Cell. Mallinckrodt Medical. April 2005.

Saha GB. *Fundamentals of Nuclear Pharmacy*. 3rd ed. New York, NY: Springer-Verlag; 1992.

7. ANSWER: B. The HVL is the amount of thickness of a material needed to reduce the exposure to half.

One layer will reduce to 2.5 mR.
Two layers will reduce to 1.25 mR.
Three layers will reduce to 0.625 mR.

The use of inverse square law $I_1 (d_2)^2 = I_2 (d_1)^2$, where I_1 = initial radiation exposure rate at distance d_1 from the source and I_2 = radiation exposure rate at distance d_2.

REFERENCE:

Early PJ, Sodee DB. *Principles and Practice of Nuclear Medicine.* St. Louis, MO: Mosby; 1985.

8. ANSWER: D. All possession, use, and disposal of radioactive material are controlled by the NRC.

REFERENCE:

Nuclear Regulatory Commission (NRC). Code of Federal Regulations, Title 10, Part 19, 20 and Part 35 for medical use.

9. ANSWER: D. Areas not under the control of the licensee and areas where a person receives <2 mrem per hour do not require posting.

REFERENCE:

Code of Federal Regulation Title 10 (NRC), Part 20.1903.

10. ANSWER: D. NRC regulation states that when an individual could receive a dose > 500 rads per hour at 1 m from the source, the area should have the Caution: High Radiation Area sign posted.

REFERENCE:

Nuclear Regulatory Commission (NRC), Code of Federal Regulation, Title 10, Part 20.1003 and 20.1902.

11. ANSWER: B. Radioactive signs are not required where radioactive materials are handled for <8 hours and are under constant observation, and in rooms where sealed sources are stored and the exposure doesn't exceed 5 mrem per hour at 1 m. Restricted areas are those to which access is limited by the licensee for the purpose of protecting individuals against unnecessary risks from exposure to radiation and radioactive materials. Usually, the hot lab, imaging room(s), and thyroid uptake room are considered restricted areas. Unrestricted areas are those areas to which access is neither limited nor controlled by the licensee.

REFERENCE:

NRC Regulation 10 Code of Federal Regulation, Title 10, Part 20.1003.

12. ANSWER: C. The transportation index of a package having radioactive materials is to be measured at a distance of 1 m from the surface.

REFERENCE:

Transportation regulation Code of Federal Regulations, Title 49, Part 172.403 and 172.436-440.

13. ANSWER: C. All of these instruments can be used to measure radiation, but the well counter is the most sensitive and practical for measuring the swipes that are used to test packages delivered to a nuclear laboratory. It is a solid scintillation counter and is very sensitive to low levels of radioactivity.

The dose calibrator is used routinely to measure radiotracer doses prior to being injected into the patient. An ionization chamber is a gas-filled enclosure between two conducting electrodes that can be used to measure gases, liquids, or solids. Geiger counters are used to detect ionizing radiation (usually beta particles and gamma rays, but certain models can detect alpha particles). An inert gas-filled tube (usually helium, neon, or argon with halogens added) briefly conducts electricity when a particle or photon of radiation makes the gas conductive. The tube amplifies this conduction by a cascade effect and outputs a current pulse, which is then often displayed by a needle or lamp and/or audible.

REFERENCE:

Saha GB. *Physics and Radiobiology of Nuclear Medicine.* 3rd ed. New York, NY: Springer-Verlag; 1993.

14. ANSWER: C. Since the patient is undergoing exercise stress, caffeine abstention is not required. Caffeine abstention is required for 12 to 24 hours when patients are scheduled to undergo dipyridamole, adenosine, or regadenoson pharmacologic stress. Caffeine may interfere with the vasodilatory effects of these drugs and lower overall accuracy by decreasing sensitivity. Beta-blockers and nitrates taken prior to stress will decrease the detection of ischemia. They should be held 12 to 24 hours prior to testing. Thallium-201 will contaminate breast milk and, due to the 72-hour half-life, will expose the infant to unnecessary radiation. Radionuclide stress testing in such patients should be delayed if possible until the patient stops breast-feeding or alternative methods of testing are considered.

REFERENCE:

Nuclear regulatory commission, Consolidated Guidance About Materials Licenses (NUREG-1556), Volume 9, Appendix U.

15. ANSWER: A. Photographic film badges consist of a holder and a radiation-sensitive film. They are used for monitoring cumulative whole-body exposure to ionizing radiation. They record both high and low radiation levels and are generally worn on the torso outside of clothing. In some circumstances, they may be worn underneath a protective lead shield to record the actual exposure to critical organs. Thermoluminescent material may in some cases be used in place of photographic films to measure whole-body exposure.

Thermoluminescent ring badges are used to measure the amount of exposure received by the hands and consist of an inorganic crystal held in a hand ring device.

A survey meter and Geiger counter are handheld devices used to measure contamination.

REFERENCES:

Nuclear Regulatory commission (NRC), Code of Federal Regulation, Title 10, Part 20.1502.
Saha GB. *Fundamentals of Nuclear Pharmacy.* 3rd ed. New York, NY: Springer-Verlag; 1992.

16. ANSWER: A. The NRC limits a radiation occupational worker to receive a total whole-body dose of 5 rem per year. It is measured in quarterly intervals so that individuals getting high rates can be identified and corrective actions taken to limit further exposure in order to avoid exceeding the yearly total. Specific organ limits include 15 rems to the eyes and 50 rems to the extremities.

REFERENCE:

Nuclear Regulatory Commission (NRC), Code of Federal Regulation, Title 10, Part 20.1201.

17. ANSWER: C. Some radioactive materials may be eliminated through the urine or feces but usually in small quantities. When released into sewage, they are diluted and do not pose a risk to patients or the public. For radionuclides used in nuclear cardiology procedures, there is minimal excretion. All of the other forms of radioactivity listed, unused patient doses and contaminated materials, should not be released directly into the sewage system. They should be allowed to decay for 10 half-lives and then disposed in the same manner used for nonradioactive materials.

Sealed radioactive sources usually have very long half-lives, and special precautions must be taken for disposal.

REFERENCE:

Nuclear Regulatory commission (NRC), Code of Federal Regulation Title 10, Art 20, Subpart K—Waste Disposal (20.2001).

18. ANSWER: A. In accordance with the ALARA (as low as reasonable achievable) principles, the NRC requires that daily surveys be performed with a survey instrument at the end of each day. Less frequent surveys would fail to detect unsafe radiation use practices that may result in unnecessary radiation exposure to patients, staff, or the public. Documentation that such surveys were performed is necessary.

REFERENCE:

Nuclear Regulatory Commission (NRC), Code of Federal Regulation Title 10, Part 20 and Part 35.70.

19. ANSWER: D. Dry paper towels or a stiff brush are best used as the initial step in decontamination of solid radioactive materials. Using hot water opens the skin pores and allows more radioactivity to be absorbed into the dermal layers. Lukewarm water with soap is best for removal of contamination.

REFERENCE:

Christian PE, Waterstram-Rich K. *Nuclear Medicine and PET/CT: Technology and Techniques.* 6th ed. St. Louis, MO: Mosby/Elsevier; 2007.

20. ANSWER: C. The dose to the embryo/fetus shall not exceed more than 500 mrem from occupational exposure for a declared pregnant worker. To monitor this occupational dose, a separate radiation film badge is issued and worn on the fetal area. Pregnant employees need to be counseled on appropriate radiation safety measures and duties without radiation exposure considered. The risks to the fetus are highest during the first trimester.

REFERENCE:

Nuclear Regulatory Commission (NRC), Code of Federal Regulation, Title 10, Part 20.1208.

21. ANSWER: D. Total exposure is directly proportional to the time of exposure. Shielding with the highest possible density material reduces radiation exposure by the process of attenuation; for gamma radiation, higher atomic number materials should be used. Distance alone reduces the exposure and varies inversely as the square of the distance from the source to the exposure point, that is, the greater the distance, the less the exposure.

REFERENCE:

Nuclear Regulatory Commission (NRC) Regulation, Federal Regulation Title 10, Part 20.1003 ALARA (acronym for "as low as is reasonably achievable").

22. ANSWER: B.
$$1/T_e = 1/T_b + 1/T_p$$
$$1/3 = 1/T_b + 1/6$$
$$T_b = 6 \text{ hours}$$

REFERENCES:

Heller GV, Hendel RC, Mann A, Eds. *Nuclear Cardiology: Technical Applications.* McGraw-Hill; 2009.
Package Insert Tc99m Sestamibi, Mallinckrodt Medical, Inc.

23. ANSWER: B. The DOT and the NRC have set limits on the amount of radiation that can be detected at the surface and at 1 m from a package containing radioactivity. The categories are listed in Table 2-1. The labeling category will determine the shielding requirements.

TABLE 2-1 Limits for DOT Labeling			
	White I	Yellow II	Yellow III
Surface (mR/h)	<0.5	>0.5, <50	>50, <200
At 1 m	<1.0	>1.0, <10	

REFERENCES:

Nuclear Regulatory Commission Regulation, Code of Federal Regulation Title 10, Part 71.
U.S. Department of Transportation Regulation, Code of Federal Regulation Title 49, Part 173.

24. ANSWER: C. The time delay after injection of a technetium-99m perfusion agent is to allow clearance from the liver and maximize the myocardial uptake. Immediately and 15 minutes after a resting or pharmacologic stress injection, there is too much liver activity present to see the inferior wall of the heart without contamination. At 30 to 60 minutes, there is adequate liver clearance to visualize the inferior wall. By 2 hours, the liver will have cleared, but there is a greater probability of having loops of bowel adjacent to the heart and there is greater decay of the radioactivity in the heart.

REFERENCE:

Henzlova M, Cerqueria MD, Hansen CL, et al. ASNC imaging guidelines for nuclear cardiology procedures: stress protocols and tracers. *J Nucl Cardiol.* 2009;16:331.

25. ANSWER: A. The rest dose should be approximately one-third the stress dose with some variation introduced by the length of time between the two studies. If the interval between studies is short, the stress requires a higher dose, and if it is long, the full three times greater dose may not be needed due to decay of the resting injection. With 1:3 dosing, the higher stress dose overcomes the smaller rest dose so that the stress images have less residual activity from the rest study. If the rest dose is high, the stress dose will need to be three times higher, and this will give the patient an unacceptably high level of radiation. If a lower dose is used for stress without enough time between the injections, there will be residual activity from the rest study that can underestimate the amount of ischemia present. The rest imaging can be started 30 to 60 minutes postinjection, and the stress imaging started 10 to 20 minutes after exercise stress and 30 to 60 after pharmacologic stress.

REFERENCE:

Henzlova MJ, Duvall WL, Einstein AJ, et al. ASNC imaging guidelines for SPECT nuclear cardiology procedures: stress, protocols, and tracers. *J Nucl Cardiol.* 2009;23:606–639. doi:10.1007/s12350-015-0387-x. https://www.asnc.org/files/Guidelines%20and%20Quality/ASNC%20SPECT%20ProtocolsTracers %20Guidelines2016.pdf

26. ANSWER: B. Technetium-99m–labeled agents have improved SPECT imaging characteristics compared to thallium-201 due to the higher photon energy (140 KeV vs. 60–80 KeV), which has less total attenuation and the shorter half-life (6 hours vs. 72 hours) allowing administration of a much higher dose but less total body radiation.

The liver and GI activity associated with the technetium-99m tracers has proven to be a major problem due to scatter, scaling or normalizing problems, and ramp filter artifacts associated with filtered back projection during reconstruction.

The extraction fraction across the coronary bed is actually lower for both technetium-99m agents in comparison to thallium-201, and this raised theoretical concerns regarding lower sensitivity for technetium-99m during the much higher coronary flow rates achieved with vasodilator pharmacologic stress.

27. ANSWER: A. Various methods have been utilized for attenuation correction including a radioactive line source (gadolinium) and x-ray–based techniques (computed tomography). Both methods create a patient-specific tissue attenuation map that is used to correct for the loss of counts due to differences in the amount and type of tissue between the heart and the detector. Attenuation correction remains a vendor-specific tool with no uniform standards established by industry or professional medical societies. When applied correctly, attenuation correction reduces soft tissue–related defects and specificity increases, so fewer studies are read as abnormal due to attenuation that may frequently be misinterpreted as a prior infarction.

28. ANSWER: A. Attenuation-corrected gender maps are not different between males and females. Attenuation correction improves the normalcy rate to a larger extent than does quantitative analysis alone. Therefore, the specificity of a positive finding is higher in images interpreted in the setting of attenuation correction.

REFERENCES:

Grossman GB, Garcia EV, Bateman TM, et al. Quantitative Tc-99m sestamibi attenuation-corrected SPECT: development and multicenter trial validation of myocardial perfusion stress gender-independent normal database in an obese population. *J Nucl Cardiol.* 2004;11:263.

Hendel RC, Corbett JR, Cullom SJ, et al. The value and practice of attenuation correction for myocardial perfusion SPECT imaging: a joint position statement from the American Society of Nuclear Cardiology and the Society of Nuclear Medicine. *J Nucl Cardiol.* 2002;9:135.

Thompson RC, Heller GV, Johnson LL, et al. Value of attenuation correction on ECG-gated SPECT myocardial perfusion imaging related to body mass index. *J Nucl Cardiol.* 2005;12:195.

29. ANSWER: C. Title 10 of the Code of Federal Regulations, Part 35, Section 35.204 (10 CFR 35.204), "Permissible molybdenum-99, strontium-82, and strontium-85 concentrations," of 0.15 kilobecquerel of Mo-99 per megabecquerel of Tc-99m (0.15 microcurie [μCi] of Mo-99 per millicurie [mCi] of technetium-99m [Tc-99m]).

30. ANSWER: B. NRC regulates the safe use and handling of all radioactive materials. Al ions limits are recommended by United States Pharmacopeia (USP-XXIII)—Limits are 10 μg/mL of eluate.

31. ANSWER: B. NRC regulations Title 10 of the Code of Federal Regulations, Section 20.1906 "Procedures for receiving and opening packages."

The licensee shall perform the monitoring required by paragraph (b) of this section as soon as practical after receipt of the package, but not later than 3 hours after the package is received at the licensee's facility if it is received during the licensee's normal working hours, or not later than 3 hours from the beginning of the next working day if it is received after working hours.

32. ANSWER: A. NCRP (National Council on Radiation Protection) Report No. 160, Ionizing Radiation Exposure of the Population of the United States.

NCRP report 160 emphasized that the average exposure to members of public in the United States has increased from 360 mrem (3.6 mSv) in 1980s to 620 mrem (6.2 mSv) in 2006. This increase is from medical uses of radiation from nuclear medicine and x-ray, predominately from diagnostic CT.

33. ANSWER: C. Title 10 of the Code of Federal Regulations, Part 35, Section 35.92, Decay-in-storage.

A licensee may hold by-product material with a physical half-life of less than or equal to 120 days for decay-in-storage before disposal without regard to its radioactivity. The lab should monitor by-product material at the surface before disposal and determines that its radioactivity cannot be distinguished from the background radiation level with an appropriate radiation detection survey meter set on its most sensitive scale and with no interposed shielding.

CHAPTER 3

Nuclear Cardiology Diagnostic Tests and Procedures/Protocols/ Artifacts

Wael A. Jaber

QUESTIONS

1. Which of the following is an indication for performing pharmacologic stress in lieu of a treadmill test for single photon emission computed tomography myocardial perfusion imaging (SPECT MPI)?

    A. Severe symptomatic peripheral vascular disease

    B. Chronotropic incompetence

    C. Left bundle-branch block (LBBB)

    D. Neurologic and muscular disorders

    E. All of the choices

2. Which of the following is not a contraindication to performing a pharmacologic stress testing with adenosine?

    A. Pentoxifylline

    B. Caffeinated foods or beverages <12 hours prior to stress test

    C. Severe obstructive lung disease with ongoing wheezing

    D. Dipyridamole or aminophylline <24 hours prior to stress test

    E. Second/third-degree atrioventricular (AV) block or sick sinus syndrome without a pacemaker

3. In which of the patients with an ST elevation acute myocardial infarction (AMI) is there an appropriate role for SPECT MPI?

A. Stable patients who have undergone coronary angiography and percutaneous intervention (PCI)

B. Decompensated congestive heart failure (CHF) patients with life-threatening arrhythmias and hemodynamic instability

C. Stable patients who have undergone successful reperfusion and coronary angiography

D. Stable patients scheduled for coronary angiography

E. Stable patients prior to discharge who are not scheduled to undergo cardiac catheterization

4. A 49-year-old woman is being evaluated for atypical chest pain. She had an acute myocardial infarction 2 years ago and received a bare metal stent to the mid-left anterior descending. After consulting her primary care physician, she is concerned about the use of SPECT MPI. Which of the following statements regarding SPECT MPI in women is/are correct?

A. Women have smaller hearts, which improves image quality and accuracy.

B. Breast attenuation is not reduced by using technetium-99m radiopharmaceuticals.

C. SPECT diagnostic specificity in women is above 90%.

D. The best use of the test is in women with intermediate to high pretest likelihood for coronary artery disease (CAD).

E. Positron emission tomography (PET) has the same diagnostic accuracy as SPECT in women.

5. An elderly female patient with renal impairment and chest pain is referred for SPECT MPI. Which of the following statements is true?

A. The more severe the renal dysfunction, the lower the likelihood of an abnormal SPECT.

B. Mortality is increased in patients with a normal MPI and moderate to severe renal dysfunction.

C. Thallium-201 SPECT stress testing is not effective in renal-impaired patients for predicting high risk of a major cardiac event.

D. Patients who undergo SPECT imaging prior to transplant are found to have ischemia in up to 10%, and they have a high adverse cardiac event rate.

6. Technetium-99m–labeled perfusion tracers are most commonly used to assess resting and stress myocardial perfusion. Studies have shown that the administration of nitrates prior to the resting injection images results in which of the following?

   A. Improves reader's ability to detect viable myocardium in severely hypoperfused segments

   B. Improves overall delivery of tracer to the myocardium and therefore improves the quality of the images

   C. Interferes with interpretation of the stress images

   D. Is of no value, since technetium-99m–labeled agents do not redistribute

   E. None of the choices

7. Which of the following statements regarding the general sensitivity and specificity for detection of CAD of various cardiac stress testing imaging methods is true?

   A. PET is most sensitive but least specific.

   B. SPECT MPI is more sensitive and specific compared to exercise electrocardiogram (ECG).

   C. Stress echocardiography is more sensitive but less specific than SPECT.

   D. The sensitivity and specificity of all tests are independent of the population studied.

8. Exercise SPECT MPI is the best initial test in which of the following situations?

   A. A 27-year-old female patient with sharp chest pain, no risk factors, a normal resting ECG, and able to exercise

   B. A 72-year-old male with atypical chest pain, diabetes and hypertension, left ventricular hypertrophy (LVH), and able to exercise

   C. A 69-year-old male with atypical chest pain, new-onset atrial fibrillation, an ECG with 2-mm ST depression, and unable to exercise

   D. A symptomatic 76-year-old female patient with increasing typical chest pain, a three-vessel coronary bypass surgery 2 years ago, a normal resting ECG, and able to exercise

9. Failure to achieve 85% of the maximal age-predicted heart rate during SPECT imaging may reduce the diagnostic performance by which of the following?

    A. Reducing the size and severity of the perfusion defects

    B. Interfering with the acquisition of ECG-gated images

    C. Not allowing enough time for tracer uptake

    D. Lowering the normalcy rate of the test

10. Which of the following is an advantage of dual-isotope SPECT MPI?

    A. Flexibility of performing 1-day stress/rest, rest/stress, or 2-day sequence

    B. Existence of validated attenuation correction algorithms for thallium-201 but not technetium-99

    C. Improved efficiency in the nuclear cardiology laboratory

    D. Easier interpretation of artifacts

11. Which of the following variables is not part of the Duke Treadmill Score?

    A. Anginal chest pain

    B. Chronotropic incompetence

    C. Magnitude of ST segment changes

    D. Exercise time

12. Which of the following is not a contraindication for SPECT stress MPI?

    A. Decompensated CHF

    B. Unstable angina

    C. Stable post–myocardial infarction

    D. Critical valvular heart disease

13. Relative to treadmill exercise ECG testing in women, SPECT MPI does which of the following?

    A. Is comparable in sensitivity and specificity

    B. Improves the specificity

    C. Improves the specificity but compromises the sensitivity

    D. Improves the sensitivity but compromises the specificity

14. Which of the following does not result in poor SPECT quality or creation of artifacts?

    A. Body size and habitus

    B. LVH

    C. Patient gender

    D. Patient position relative to the camera

15. In a male patient undergoing SPECT MPI, which of the following is least likely to cause an artifact?

    A. Abdominal protuberance

    B. Anterior chest attenuation related to obesity

    C. Shifting breast artifact

    D. Elevated diaphragm

16. Breast attenuation is likely to create SPECT artifacts resulting in which of the following?

    A. Decreased sensitivity in the right coronary artery (RCA) territory

    B. Decreased specificity in the RCA territory

    C. Decreased sensitivity in the left anterior descending (LAD) artery territory

    D. Decreased specificity in the LAD territory

17. All of the following are measures employed to limit or recognize attenuation artifacts in SPECT MPI except:

    A. Utilizing higher-energy pharmaceutical.

    B. Reviewing rotating projection images.

    C. Performing quantitative analysis.

    D. Using pharmacologic in place of exercise stress.

18. Quantitative analysis of SPECT MPI has been used to help differentiate attenuation artifacts from true perfusion defects. Comparison of a given patient to which of the following normal databases gives the best specificity?

    A. Age matched

    B. Gender matched

    C. Weight matched

    D. Risk factor matched

19. Prone imaging improves SPECT MPI accuracy because it allows recognition of which of the following?

    A. Diaphragmatic attenuation

    B. Patient motion

    C. Breast attenuation

    D. Residual liver activity

20. Which of the following is a true statement about gated SPECT MPI?

    A. It has a very high spatial and temporal resolution compared to echocardiographic methods.

    B. It is generated from the best cardiac cycles during image acquisition.

    C. It improves specificity and reader confidence in the SPECT interpretation.

    D. The ejection fraction measurements can help in the diagnosis of diastolic dysfunction.

21. Which of the following maneuvers is most likely to eliminate liver retention with technetium-99 radiotracers and improve image quality?

    A. Having the patient drink two 8-ounce glasses of water and imaging immediately after pharmacologic stress

    B. Having the patient drink 4-ounce glasses of a carbonated drink and imaging immediately after pharmacologic stress

    C. Waiting 45 minutes before imaging following pharmacologic stress

    D. Switching the patient from exercise to pharmacologic stress

22. Which of the following is/are the most appropriate reason(s) for using pharmacologic stress testing?

    A. Peripheral vascular disease limiting exertion

    B. Presence of left bundle-branch block (LBBB) or pacemaker

    C. Failure to achieve target heart rate with dynamic exercise

    D. All of the choices

23. Although vasodilators are generally preferred for pharmacologic stress SPECT MPI, in which of the following situations is dobutamine the most appropriate stress agent?

    A. Patients taking beta-blockers

    B. Patients who are in atrial fibrillation

    C. Patients in whom a higher-sensitivity SPECT study is desired

    D. Patients who are being treated with theophylline

24. Which of the following is the most appropriate explanation for why dipyridamole, regadenoson, and adenosine are effective pharmacologic SPECT stress agents?

    A. Ability to increase coronary blood flow 2.4 to 4.5 times above baseline

    B. Increase in heart rate and blood pressure products

    C. Dilation of epicardial coronary vessels

    D. Dilation of critically stenosed coronary vessels

25. Which adenosine receptor induces coronary vasodilation when activated?

    A. A1

    B. A2A

    C. A2B

    D. A3

26. Which of the following is a cardiovascular effect of adenosine?

    A. Vasoconstriction

    B. Vagal-mediated bradycardia

    C. Increased adrenergic activation

    D. Bradycardia and AV block

27. Which of the following is a biologic effect of dipyridamole?

    A. It is taken up rapidly by red blood cells and endothelial cells.

    B. The biologic half-life of dipyridamole is 30 to 45 seconds.

    C. It is primarily metabolized in the liver.

    D. Due to its short half-life, it is not used in PET imaging.

28. The side effects reported with adenosine and dipyridamole are due to which of the following?

    A. Stimulation of A2A receptors

    B. Stimulation of A1, A2B, and A3 receptors

    C. Generation of metabolites

    D. Paradoxical coronary vasoconstriction

29. Which of the following is a feature of regadenoson?

    A. Shorter half-life than adenosine

    B. Selective activation of A2A receptors

    C. Longer administration time

    D. Weight-adjusted dose

30. Relative to adenosine, patients receiving regadenoson are more likely to have which of the following?

    A. Headaches

    B. Perfusion defects

    C. Lower poststress ejection fraction

    D. Higher incidence of dyspnea, flushing, and chest pain

31. Which of the following patients should not receive dipyridamole, adenosine, or regadenoson for SPECT MPI pharmacologic stress?

    A. Taking oral dipyridamole

    B. Known sick sinus syndrome

    C. Known high-degree AV block

    D. Taking Aggrenox

    E. All of the choices

32. Coronary steal is sometimes described in patients undergoing vasodilator pharmacologic SPECT and PET stress tests. When this phenomenon occurs, it is usually:

    A. Clinically silent.

    B. Associated with ST changes and/or symptoms.

    C. Related to adequate flow in the collateral circulation.

    D. Only seen in patients who had prior bypass coronary surgery.

33. Simultaneous low-level exercise is often used during vasodilator SPECT pharmacologic stress testing. The main advantage of low-level exercise is:

    A. Increased coronary vasodilation.

    B. Achieving maximal predicted heart rate.

    C. Inducing true ischemia.

    D. Reducing side effects.

34. When using vasodilators for pharmacologic SPECT or PET stress testing, which of the following statements is true?

    A. Beta-blockers, calcium channel blockers, and nitrates have no impact on the sensitivity of the test and can be continued.

    B. Beta-blockers, calcium channel blockers, and nitrates can decrease the sensitivity of the test and should be discontinued if possible 24 hours before the test.

    C. Only nitrates can decrease the sensitivity of the test.

    D. Only calcium channel blockers can decrease the sensitivity of the test.

35. In patients with chronic kidney disease undergoing pharmacologic SPECT stress testing, the following statement is true:

    A. The annual death rate with a normal scan is <1% per year.

    B. Ischemia but not scar is a predictor of mortality.

    C. Scar but not ischemia is a predictor of mortality.

    D. Both scar and ischemia are predictors of events.

36. Which of the following is the most appropriate indication for performing SPECT MPI?

    A. Low likelihood of CAD, interpretable ECG, and able to exercise

    B. Chest pain with ST elevation

    C. High pretest likelihood of disease

    D. Intermediate pretest probability of CAD

37. A 37-year-old male presents for a general health "checkup." He has no symptoms or current risk factors for CAD, but he is very concerned because his exercise partner had a stress SPECT study and was found to have ischemia and multivessel disease. Is a stress SPECT MPI an appropriate test?

    A. He is at intermediate risk for CAD and a stress SPECT is appropriate.

    B. He is at high risk for CAD and a coronary angiogram is appropriate.

    C. He is at low risk and a stress SPECT stress test is inappropriate.

    D. A SPECT stress test followed by a CT calcium score is appropriate.

38. You are seeing a 57-year-old male patient in a preventive cardiology setting. He has a body mass index (BMI) of 29 and is hypertensive. He is also known to have "abnormal cholesterol" but tells you that his cholesterol now is normal on simvastatin. He has no symptoms and exercises three times per week when he is off duty from his job as a commercial pilot. His baseline ECG shows normal sinus rhythm and 1-mm ST depression inferolaterally. Based on his presentation:

    A. You recommend aggressive risk factors modification only.

    B. You recommend aggressive risk factors modification and a stress SPECT myocardial perfusion test for risk assessment.

    C. You recommend a pharmacologic SPECT and aggressive risk factors modification.

    D. He is asymptomatic and therefore no further risk assessment is needed.

39. A 63-year-old female patient has a family history of CAD, prior tobacco use, hypertension, and diabetes. She had a normal SPECT MPI study 1.5 years earlier and was told to get a yearly SPECT for follow-up assessment. She apologizes for missing her appointment at 1 year to have the stress test done but tells you that she brought her running shoes and she is fasting and ready for the stress test today. She is overall asymptomatic and participates in a walking club with yoga 5 days/wk after work. Based on her presentation, you recommend:

    A. Proceed with stress SPECT study given her risk profile.

    B. Only a stress ECG without imaging.

    C. A coronary calcium score followed by a stress SPECT.

    D. No stress test is needed now. Continue aggressive risk factors modifications.

40. A 47-year-old female premenopausal patient who presents for preoperative risk assessment prior to laparoscopic gallbladder surgery. She has a history of hypertension that is treated with low-dose diuretic and is otherwise "healthy." She power walks five times per week without any symptoms. Her baseline ECG shows normal sinus rhythm with infrequent premature beats and otherwise is unremarkable. The anesthesiologist recommended a stress test prior to the gallbladder surgery. Your recommendation was:

    A. Proceed with surgery. Patient is at acceptable risk.

    B. Stress ECG for further risk assessment.

    C. Stress SPECT MPI given the baseline ECG.

    D. Stress echocardiogram given the baseline ECG and to avoid radiation exposure.

41. Which of the following patients is at the highest risk for serious hypotension in patients receiving regadenoson for SPECT MPI?

    A. Female patients

    B. Male patients

    C. Patients with autonomic dysfunction

    D. Patients with peripheral vascular disease

42. For symptoms occurring in >5% of patients receiving regadenoson for SPECT MPI, which of the following side effects lasts longest?

A. Dyspnea

B. Headache

C. Chest pain/discomfort

D. Dizziness

43. In patients who received an initial adenosine study and were then randomized to receive either a repeat adenosine or a regadenoson, what was the interobserver agreement rate between adenosine versus adenosine and adenosine versus regadenoson?

A. 85% to 90%

B. 30% to 35%

C. 60% to 65%

D. 50%

ANSWERS

1. ANSWER: E. Pharmacologic MPI is reserved for patients who are unable to exercise or who can exercise but fail to achieve at least 85% of the maximal age-predicted heart rate. Thus, patients with severe peripheral vascular disease and neurologic and muscular disorders have exercise limitations and patients who cannot increase their heart rates sufficiently due to chronotropic incompetence are candidates for pharmacologic stress. Patients with LBBB or electronically paced rhythms may develop a septal perfusion abnormality in the absence of septal branch or LAD disease due to decreased septal blood flow at rapid heart rates. With pharmacologic stress, the heart rate does not increase and specificity is improved. Dobutamine stress is not appropriate as it increases heart rate. In such patients, if there is an associated anterior or apical defect in addition to the septal abnormality, this is usually associated with LAD artery disease.

Patients with permanent pacing can also develop perfusion defects in the septum, inferior wall, and apex in the absence of disease and the mechanism also is related to asynchronous contraction of the myocardium.

Adenosine or dipyridamole and recently regadenoson are the pharmacologic agents of choice for patients with an LBBB or are ventricularly paced.

REFERENCE:

Skalidis EI, Kochiadakis GE, Koukouraki SI, et al. Phasic coronary flow pattern and flow reserve in patients with left bundle-branch block and normal coronary arteries. *J Am Coll Cardiol.* 1999;33:1338–1346.

2. ANSWER: A. Adenosine is a nonselective agonist that causes coronary vasodilation when it activates the A2A receptor. The other receptors (A1, A2B, and A3) when activated produce most of the side effects that include chest pain, bronchiolar constriction, mast cell degranulation (flushing), and negative chronotropic, inotropic, and dromotropic effects.

Pentoxifylline, a xanthine derivative used for intermittent claudication, can be continued prior to adenosine. Compounds such as caffeine and aminophylline bind to adenosine receptors without stimulating them but prevent the vasodilation induced by adenosine, regadenoson, or dipyridamole, which lowers sensitivity for detection of CAD. Caffeine should be held 12 to 24 hours prior to the test and aminophylline-containing compounds for 24 to 48 hours depending on the formulation. If patients are taking dipyridamole, it should be held for 24 to 48 hours. If dipyridamole has been taken orally and intravenous dipyridamole is used as a stressor, the patient already has some degree of vasodilation and the resting study will have a high baseline blood flow and the flow reserve during stress is decreased. If dipyridamole has been taken and adenosine or regadenoson are used for pharmacologic stress, their half-lives are markedly prolonged due to inhibition by dipyridamole of the bidirectional adenosine transport mechanism that is responsible for the short half-lives of these compounds.

Patients with severe obstructive lung disease with active wheezing should not undergo adenosine or dipyridamole stress testing due to the activation of the A2B/A3 receptors that produce bronchial constriction. However, American Society of Nuclear Cardiology (ASNC) recommends patients with adequately controlled obstructive lung disease can undergo an adenosine stress test and can have pretreatment with one to two puffs of albuterol or a comparable inhaler.

AV block occurs in ~7.6% of patients receiving adenosine but is very rare with dipyridamole. However, the incidence of second-degree AV block is only 4% and that of complete heart block is <1%. The presence of second- or third-degree AV block or sick sinus syndrome without a pacemaker is a contraindication to adenosine, regadenoson, or dipyridamole stress due to the activation of A1 receptors that are located in the SA, AV, atrial, and ventricular myocytes producing negative chronotropic, inotropic, and dromotropic effects.

REFERENCES:

Boger LA, Volver LL, Herstein GK, et al. Best patient preparation before and during radionuclide myocardial perfusion imaging studies. *J Nucl Cardiol.* 2006;13:98–110.

Henzlova MJ, Cerqueira MD, Mahmarian JJ, et al. Stress protocols and tracers. *J Nucl Cardiol.* 2006;13:e80–e90.

O'Keefe JH Jr, Bateman TM, Barnhart CS. Adenosine thallium-201 is superior to exercise thallium-201 for selecting coronary artery disease in patients with left bundle-branch block. *J Am Coll Cardiol.* 1999;21:1332–1338.

3. ANSWER: E. E is a class I indication with level of evidence B. In patients unable to exercise who are not scheduled to undergo cardiac catheterization, dipyridamole, adenosine, or regadenoson MPI prior to or early after discharge to look for inducible ischemia is indicated since the results can further risk stratify the patient and help the clinician select the most appropriate treatment strategy.

All of the other patients have had coronary angiography and treatment and are stable, are very unstable and need coronary angiography, or are scheduled for coronary angiography. In such patients, SPECT MPI will not provide further diagnostic or management information. In patients with coronary angiography who had intermediate lesions that need to be assessed, testing once patients have recovered may be useful.

REFERENCE:

Antman EM. 2004 update: a report of the ACC/AHA Task Force on Practice Guidelines. (Committee on Management of Acute Myocardial Infarction). Available at http://www.acc.org

4. ANSWER: D. Small left ventricular chamber size adversely affects image quality and diagnostic accuracy especially if using thallium-201 SPECT MPI. Women have smaller hearts than men, which diminishes accuracy.

Breast attenuation can produce anterior wall defects that may mimic an LAD distribution infarction. Technetium-99 agents with ECG gating have less attenuation and give better gated images than thallium-201, which improves accuracy by improving specificity.

Specificity for diagnosing CAD is reduced to 65% to 70% due to breast tissue artifact but can be improved to 85% to 90% range when clinicians integrate the rotating projection images, wall motion, and attenuation correction.

The AHA recommends MPI in men or women if they have intermediate to high pretest likelihood for CAD where the test is likely to reclassify patients into to a high- or low-risk category.

PET has higher diagnostic accuracy than SPECT in women with improved accuracy by more successfully addressing such problems as breast attenuation, obesity, and small heart size.

REFERENCES:

Mieres JH, Shaw LJ, Arai A, et al.; Cardiac Imaging Committee, Council on Clinical Cardiology, and the Cardiovascular Imaging and Intervention Committee, Council on Cardiovascular Radiology and Intervention, American Heart Association. Role of noninvasive testing in the clinical evaluation of women with suspected coronary artery disease: Consensus statement from the Cardiac Imaging Committee, Council on Clinical Cardiology, and the Cardiovascular Imaging and Intervention Committee, Council on Cardiovascular Radiology and Intervention, American Heart Association. *Circulation.* 2005;111(5):682–696.

Sampson UK, Dorbala S, Limaye A, et al. Diagnostic accuracy of rubidium-82 myocardial perfusion imaging with hybrid positron emission tomography/computed tomography in the detection of coronary artery disease. *J Am Coll Cardiol.* 2007;49(10):1052–1058.

5. ANSWER: D. The presence of renal dysfunction predisposes to accelerated atherogenesis and increased cardiovascular event risk. Al-Mallah MH demonstrated that mortality almost doubles in patients with moderate or severe renal impairment (GFR < 60 mL/min/1.73 m^2) in the presence of an abnormal stress SPECT MPI.

Dahan evaluated the utility of SPECT imaging in hemodialysis patients and found that the negative predictive value is 91% after 2.87 years of follow-up for major cardiovascular events and that sensitivity and specificity for detection of disease are similar to a population not on dialysis.

Although a small study, Dussol evaluated 97 patients prior to renal transplantation and found that 10% had inducible ischemia on SPECT and that these patients had increased adverse event rates.

There is a significant interaction between ischemia on SPECT MPI and renal function. The more severe the renal dysfunction, the higher the probability of having an abnormal SPECT study, and the more severe the ischemia. There are many postulated mechanisms for this relationship that are beyond the scope of this review.

REFERENCES:

Al-Mallah MH, Hachamovitch R, Dorbala S, et al. Incremental prognostic value of myocardial perfusion imaging in patients referred to stress single-photon emission computed tomography with renal dysfunction. *Circ Cardiovasc Imaging.* 2009;2:429–436.

Dahan M, Viron BM, Faraggi M, et al. Diagnostic accuracy and prognostic value of combined dipyridamole-exercise thallium imaging in hemodialysis patients. *Kidney Int.* 1998;54:255–262.

Dussol B, Bonnet JL, Sampol J, et al. Prognostic value of inducible myocardial ischemia in predicting cardiovascular events after renal transplantation. *Kidney Int.* 2004;66:1633–1639.

6. ANSWER: A. The use of nitrates in conjunction with rest technetium-99m sestamibi SPECT MPI has been shown to improve detection of viable myocardium, similar to the results observed with thallium-201. Compared with resting technetium-99m sestamibi studies alone, nitrate-enhanced SPECT has a greater ability to predict improvement of regional function after revascularization and to provide important prognostic information. The demonstration of "defect reversibility" on nitrate-enhanced compared to resting images may have better accuracy than either technique alone.

7. ANSWER: B. Although evaluated in a smaller number of studies than SPECT, stress echocardiography, and the exercise ECG, cardiac PET has the highest sensitivity and specificity of currently available noninvasive modalities. SPECT has a reported higher sensitivity and lower specificity in comparison to stress echocardiography. In comparison to the stress ECG, SPECT has both a higher sensitivity and specificity. In all the published studies for any given modality, the population under study has a major influence on the accuracy of the studies. Imaging studies performed in a very low-risk population are likely to have more false positives as the prevalence of disease will be lower, and this results in lower test specificity. Similarly, when the prevalence of CAD is very high, negative studies have a higher probability of being false negatives resulting in a lower sensitivity. It is also very important to define the gold standard to determine whether an imaging study is positive or negative. Studies using patients clinically referred for coronary angiography before or after an imaging study suffer from posttest referral bias. That is, patients with a normal imaging study are not as likely to be referred for coronary angiography. Published studies estimate a referral bias of ~3%. This posttest referral bias may result in a lower specificity and may increase the reported sensitivity.

REFERENCES:

Fleischmann KE, Hunink MG, Kuntz KM, et al. Exercise echocardiography or exercise SPECT imaging? A meta-analysis of diagnostic test performance. *JAMA.* 1998;280:913.

Garber AM, Solomon NA. Cost-effectiveness of alternative test strategies for the diagnosis of coronary artery disease. *Ann Intern Med.* 1999;130:719.

Marwick T, D'Hondt AM, Baudhuin T, et al. Optimal use of dobutamine stress for the detection and evaluation of coronary artery disease: combination with echocardiography or scintigraphy, or both? *J Am Coll Cardiol.* 1993;22:159.

8. ANSWER: B. In a female patient with a low pretest probability for CAD who has a normal baseline ECG and is capable of exercising, SPECT MPI is not indicated and a stress ECG is the best initial test. A patient with an intermediate probability of CAD and LVH on the baseline ECG is the best candidate for exercise stress SPECT. The ECG alone would not be diagnostic and imaging is required. In patients with an intermediate probability of CAD who are unable to exercise, pharmacologic stress SPECT is the best test and not exercise. In a patient with known CAD and typical symptoms, the probability of graft stenosis or progression of native CAD is sufficiently high that coronary angiography may be the best initial test.

9. ANSWER: A. Failure to achieve 85% of the maximal age-predicted heart rated during exercise stress may not cause enough of an increase in coronary blood flow to create sufficient flow heterogeneity between areas of the myocardium supplied by an artery with a critical stenosis and those with nonstenosed arteries when the radiotracer is injected. Although the presence of clinical endpoints such as typical anginal symptoms or profound ECG changes of ischemia are reasons to inject the radiotracer at a submaximal heart rate, tracer administration without these endpoints or the target heart rate will result in the absence or a smaller degree of inducible ischemia and a lower sensitivity.

REFERENCES:

Heller GV, Ahmed I, Tilikemeier PL, et al. Influence of exercise intensity on the presence, distribution, size of thallium-201 defects. *Am Heart J.* 1992;123:909.

Iskandrian AS, Heo J, Kong B, et al. Effect of exercise level on the ability of thallium-201 tomographic imaging in detecting coronary artery disease: analysis of 461 patients. *J Am Coll Cardiol.* 1989;14:1477.

10. ANSWER: C. All but choice C is advantage of a technetium-99 single-isotope imaging strategy. Dual-isotope studies can be performed in a much shorter time period as there is no waiting for liver clearance as is required with the technetium-99 tracers and the studies can be completed in a much shorter time interval. The radiation exposure of dual-isotope imaging is 25 to 30 mSv, while single-isotope rest/stress technetium-99 imaging is ~8 to 15 mSv. Attenuation correction to determine attenuation artifact has been validated for technetium-based imaging agents but not thallium-201.

REFERENCE:

Thompson RC, Cullom SJ. Issues regarding radiation dosage of cardiac nuclear and radiography procedures. *J Nucl Cardiol.* 2006;13:19.

11. ANSWER: B. Although chronotropic incompetence has been shown to predict future cardiac events, it is not a variable that was included in the original Duke Treadmill Score.

REFERENCES:

Mark DB, Hlatky MA, Harrell FE Jr, et al. Exercise treadmill score for predicting prognosis in coronary artery disease. *Ann Intern Med.* 1987;106(6):793–800.

Mark DB, Shaw L, Harrell FE Jr, et al. Prognostic value of a treadmill exercise score in outpatients with suspected coronary artery disease. *N Engl J Med.* 1991;325(12):849–853.

12. ANSWER: C. Uncompensated CHF unstable angina and critical valvular heart disease are contraindications for exercise stress testing.

Stable post–myocardial infarction patients can be evaluated with pharmacologic stress to assess prognosis and residual ischemia and need for coronary angiography.

13. ANSWER: B. SPECT improves specificity without compromising sensitivity in the detection of CAD in women compared to exercise ECG stress testing alone.

REFERENCE:

Mieres JH, Shaw LJ, Hendel RC, et al. A report of the American Society of Nuclear Cardiology Task Force on Women and Heart Disease (writing group on perfusion imaging in women). *J Nucl Cardiol.* 2003;10:95.

14. ANSWER: B. SPECT MPI without attenuation correction is adversely influenced by the presence of different tissue densities and the distance between the heart and the gamma camera. Camera distance from the patient, whether due to obesity or poor positioning at the time of acquisition, results in lower counts and poor quality studies. Breast size, density and position, and diaphragmatic position and thickness all cause attenuation resulting in low counts in the covered portions of the myocardium and the appearance of less tracer uptake in the presence of normal coronary blood supply. LVH may improve count statistics, which results in better-quality images with the risk of hiding small areas of ischemia.

15. ANSWER: C. Abdominal protuberance due to obesity or ascites can cause elevation of the diaphragm and greater inferior wall attenuation and the need to position the gamma camera head further from the patient, which will lower total counts and give poor image quality. Chest wall obesity also requires positioning the gamma camera head further from the patient, and there is greater tissue density to cause attenuation. Although morbidly obese male patients may have substantial gynecomastia, the breast tissue is unlikely to shift in position between the rest and stress studies as is commonly seen in females who have pendulous breasts. An elevated diaphragm for whatever reason is likely to cause diaphragmatic attenuation.

16. ANSWER: D. Breast attenuation artifacts are seen in 40% of myocardial perfusion images in women. These artifacts are often present in the anterior wall leading to a lower specificity to correctly diagnose CAD in the LAD territory.

17. ANSWER: D. The use of technetium-99–radiolabeled perfusion agents results in less attenuation and scatter and gives higher-quality images than thallium-201. Review of the rotating projection images in cine format allows identification of the position of the diaphragm and breasts and estimation of the movement of the heart in the vertical and horizontal planes. Using gender-matched normal files for quantitative analysis helps to eliminate attenuation artifact. The type of stress does not influence attenuation while the higher background usually seen with pharmacologic stress results in poor image quality.

18. ANSWER: B. Normal databases are usually matched for type of protocol, form of stress, and the type of agent. Of the variables listed, gender-matched normal files improve specificity most by accounting for differences in the amount of breast attenuation. Age, weight, and risk factors are useful to give a pretest probability of disease but do not help with artifact recognition.

19. ANSWER: A. Prone imaging (patient lies on abdomen) provides greater separation between the heart and the diaphragm, so there is less inferior wall attenuation in comparison to a supine image (patient lays on back). Patients are usually imaged both prone and supine and a comparison is made. Most available normal files are for supine imaging. Patient motion, breast attenuation, and residual liver activity can be seen on both the prone and supine images.

20. ANSWER: C. Traditional gated SPECT has a low spatial and temporal resolution compared to echocardiographic methods. Spatial resolution varies from 14 to 16 mm and the temporal resolution is restricted to 8 or at most 16 time frames for the RR interval. Greater temporal resolution is limited by the resulting low counts in each time interval. ECG-gated SPECT is generated from all the cardiac cycles throughout the acquisition process. The gated images can help differentiate perfusion defects due to scar, which do not move or thicken, and attenuation defects that move and thicken. The ejection fraction is not a measure of diastolic function but rather systolic function. Diastolic function is not assessed by the EF but by looking at the diastolic filling curves. Eight frames do not provide enough temporal resolution to accurately measure the rapid ventricular filling period, but 16 frames have been used for diastolic analysis.

21. ANSWER: C. Both technetium-99 sestamibi and tetrofosmin are cleared from the liver in a time-dependent manner. Having the patient drink large amounts of water or small amounts of a carbonated liquid, which will release gas, will not enhance liver clearance and the recommended imaging time after pharmacologic stress or rest is 30 to 60 minutes. Imaging immediately after pharmacologic stress will result in significant liver retention. Delaying image acquisition and adding exercise to the stress tests can lead to better clearance and therefore lower liver and gastrointestinal counts.

22. ANSWER: D. All of the choices are appropriate indications for using pharmacologic stress. Inability to exercise or to achieve target heart rate is a clear reason to perform pharmacologic stress. In the presence of LBBB or an electronic ventricular-paced rhythm, septal perfusion defects maybe observed with dynamic exercise stress that lower specificity. These false positives are decreased when using pharmacologic stress.

23. ANSWER: D. Dobutamine is a stress inotropic agent that can be used for pharmacologic stress testing in patients with active airway disease or in patients being treated with theophylline. In such patients, dipyridamole, adenosine, or regadenoson may cause further airway decompensation by stimulation of adenosine A2B or A3 receptors that mediate bronchospasm. In patients taking theophylline, which blocks the adenosine receptors and is used to treat side effects induced by the vasodilators, these agents may not sufficiently augment coronary blood flow to provide a diagnostic study. Dobutamine is less useful when patients are being treated with beta-blockers as they are less likely to achieve 85% of the maximal age-predicted heart rate. Dobutamine is not preferred in patients in atrial fibrillation, and it does not have greater sensitivity over the vasodilators.

24. ANSWER: A. All of these agents act as direct or indirect vasodilators of the resistance arterioles varying from 2.4 to 4.5 times above the baseline blood depending on the agent. Regadenoson gives a more physiologic increase in blood flow relative to adenosine and dipyridamole, which give a greater response. In severely obstructed vessels, the arterioles are maximally dilated at baseline, and therefore, no significant vasodilation can be induced with these agents.

REFERENCES:

Chambers CE, Brown KA. Dipyridamole-induced ST segment depression during thallium-201 imaging in patients with coronary artery disease: angiographic and hemodynamic determinants. *J Am Coll Cardiol.* 1988;12:37.

Nishimura S, Kimball KT, Mahmarian JJ, et al. Angiographic and hemodynamic determinants of myocardial ischemia during adenosine thallium-201 scintigraphy in coronary artery disease. *Circulation.* 1993;87:1211.

25. ANSWER: B. Activation of A1 receptors causes AV conduction delay or AV nodal block. Activation of A2B and A3 receptors can mediate broncho-spasm by facilitating mast cell degranulation. Activation of adenosine A2A receptors causes coronary vasodilation. Adenosine and dipyridamole cause direct nonselective stimulator of all these receptors.

REFERENCE:

Shryock JC, Belardinelli L. Adenosine and adenosine receptors in the cardiovascular system: biochemistry, physiology, and pharmacology. *Am J Cardiol.* 1997;79:2.

26. ANSWER: D. The cardiovascular effects of adenosine include:
- Potent vasodilator
- Vagal inhibition at low doses leading to increase in heart rate
- Bradycardia and AV block at high doses
- Reduced adrenergic activity

REFERENCE:

Shryock JC, Belardinelli L. Adenosine and adenosine receptors in the cardiovascular system: biochemistry, physiology, and pharmacology. *Am J Cardiol.* 1997;79:2.

27. ANSWER: C. Dipyridamole is primarily metabolized in the liver and should be used cautiously in patients with hepatic dysfunction. The biologic half-life of dipyridamole is 30 to 45 minutes. Adenosine but not dipyridamole is rapidly taken up by red blood cells and endothelial cells, and this explains the short biologic half-life of adenosine. The longer half-life makes it a good agent for PET imaging as it does not need to be given as a continuous infusion over an extended time period.

28. ANSWER: B. Adenosine nonselectively activates the adenosine A1, A2B, and A3 receptors that are responsible for the undesirable side effects associated with pharmacologic stress. The stimulation of A2A receptors on arterial smooth muscle cells is what leads to coronary vasodilation.

29. ANSWER: B. Regadenoson is a selective A2A receptor agonist that was FDA-approved for use in SPECT MPI in 2008. It is the only FDA-approved selective A2A agonist at this time. Following a 10-second fixed bolus injection of 400 mcg over 10 seconds, it produces hyperemia of 2.5 times the baseline blood flow with rapid onset (30 seconds) for a longer period (~2 to 5 minutes) than adenosine, which permits more efficient simplified protocols. The single-dose protocol facilitates use and reduces errors due to weight-based dosing calculations. The half-life for regadenoson has an initial intravenous phase of 2 minutes and a longer intermediate phase of 30 minutes and a third phase of 2 hours.

30. ANSWER: A. ADVANCE MPI 1 and 2 randomized trials demonstrated noninferiority for regadenoson relative to adenosine for the detection of ischemia. Regadenoson-induced perfusion defects correlated closely with adenosine-induced defects. In both reports, regadenoson was associated with a decreased overall symptom score of dyspnea, flushing, and chest pain. However, regadenoson was more commonly associated with headache.

REFERENCES:

Cerqueira MD, Nguyen P, Staehr P, et al. Effects of age, gender, obesity, and diabetes on the efficacy and safety of the selective A2A agonist regadenoson versus adenosine in myocardial perfusion imaging integrated ADVANCE-MPI trial results. *JACC Cardiovasc Imaging.* 2008;1:307.

Iskandrian AE, Bateman TM, Belardinelli L, et al. Adenosine versus regadenoson comparative evaluation in myocardial perfusion imaging: results of the ADVANCE phase 3 multicenter international trial. *J Nucl Cardiol.* 2007;14:645.

Mahmarian JJ, Cerqueira MD, Iskandrian AE, et al. Regadenoson induces comparable left ventricular perfusion defects as adenosine: a quantitative analysis from the ADVANCE MPI 2 trial. *JACC Cardiovasc Imaging.* 2009;2:959.

31. ANSWER: E. These are all patient scenarios where adenosine, regadenoson, and dipyridamole should not be used in conjunction with pharmacologic stress. Patients taking oral dipyridamole, which is also one of the ingredients in Aggrenox, who receive adenosine, have increased adverse events as the half-life of adenosine is markedly increased over the normal value of <10 seconds. Even though regadenoson is a selective A2A agonist with less stimulation of the A1 receptors that cause AV nodal block, none of the adenosine-stimulating drugs should be used in patients with high-grade AV block without functioning pacemakers.

REFERENCES:

Cerqueira MD, Verani MS, Schwaiger M, et al. Safety profile of adenosine stress perfusion imaging: results from the Adenoscan Multicenter Trial Registry. *J Am Coll Cardiol.* 1994;23:384.

Lette J, Tatum JL, Fraser S, et al. Safety of dipyridamole testing in 73,806 patients: the Multicenter Dipyridamole Safety Study. *J Nucl Cardiol.* 1995;2:3.

Ranhosky A, Kempthorne-Rawson J. The safety of intravenous dipyridamole thallium myocardial perfusion imaging. Intravenous Dipyridamole Thallium Imaging Study Group. *Circulation.* 1990;81:1205.

32. ANSWER: B. Vasodilators do not significantly increase cardiac work or increase oxygen demands but may cause a coronary steal by dilating vessels with noncritical stenoses that are supplying collaterals to areas with high-grade stenosis. This may result in an intracoronary steal due to inadequate flow through the collaterals resulting in an endocardial to subepicardial steal. It is usually associated with clinical symptoms and ischemic ST changes. It can be seen in patients with severe native coronary disease or in patients post bypass surgery.

REFERENCES:

Akinboboye OO, Idris O, Chou RL, et al. Absolute quantitation of coronary steal induced by intravenous dipyridamole. *J Am Coll Cardiol.* 2001;37:109.

Nishimura S, Kimball KT, Mahmarian JJ, et al. Angiographic and hemodynamic determinants of myocardial ischemia during adenosine thallium-201 scintigraphy in coronary artery disease. *Circulation.* 1993;87:1211.

33. ANSWER: D. Vasodilators used in pharmacologic SPECT stress protocols produce a fourfold increase in coronary blood flow in normal coronaries, which is greater than that achieved with exercise or dobutamine stress. Ischemia is not a requirement to detect heterogeneity in coronary blood flow on the SPECT images. The patients usually undergo a low-level exercise without achieving target heart rate in order to minimize side effects of vasodilators and facilitate the clearance of tracer activity from the liver and gut, which results in better image quality.

REFERENCE:

Thomas GS, Miyamoto MI. Should simultaneous exercise become the standard for adenosine myocardial perfusion imaging? *Am J Cardiol.* 2004;94:3D.

34. ANSWER: B. Patients undergoing SPECT or PET MPI on maximal beta-blockers, calcium channel blockers, and nitrates can have normal perfusion studies or a significant reduction in the amount of detected ischemia in comparison to studies performed while off these medications. Thus, for studies performed to diagnose the presence or absence of CAD, these medications need to be discontinued for 24 to 48 hours depending on the formulation. There may be some justification to test patients with known ischemia to see how well medical or interventional therapy has reduced the amount of inducible ischemia present.

REFERENCES:

Bottcher M, Refsgaard J, Madsen MM, et al. Effect of antianginal medication on resting myocardial perfusion and pharmacologically induced hyperemia. *J Nucl Cardiol.* 2003;10:345.

Sharir T, Rabinowitz B, Livschitz S, et al. Underestimation of extent and severity of coronary artery disease by dipyridamole stress thallium-201 single-photon emission computed tomographic myocardial perfusion imaging in patients taking antianginal drugs. *J Am Coll Cardiol.* 1998;31:1540.

Taillefer R, Ahlberg AW, Masood Y, et al. Acute beta-blockade reduces the extent and severity of myocardial perfusion defects with dipyridamole Tc-99m sestamibi SPECT imaging. *J Am Coll Cardiol.* 2003;42:1475.

35. ANSWER: D. With a normal SPECT scan, the annual cardiac death rate is 2.7% when chronic kidney disease is present; with no chronic kidney disease and a normal test, the annual cardiac death rate was significantly lower (0.8%). Patients with chronic kidney disease and scar have an annual event rate of 5.7%. Patients with chronic kidney disease and ischemia have an annual event rate of 11%.

REFERENCE:

Hakeem A, Bhatti S, Dillie KS, et al. Predictive value of myocardial perfusion single-photon emission computed tomography and the impact of renal function on cardiac death. *Circulation.* 2008;118:2540.

36. ANSWER: D. Low-risk patients who can exercise and have a normal baseline ECG should undergo an ECG stress test. In a patient with an ST elevation acute coronary syndrome, imaging will not impact management and may delay initiation of appropriate therapy. In patients with a high pretest likelihood of disease, referral for a diagnostic and possible interventional coronary angiogram may be the most appropriate initial test. It is in the intermediate-probability patient that imaging may help to stratify patients into high- or low-risk categories in order to determine management (Table 3-1).

TABLE 3-1	Detection of CAD: Symptomatic	
Indication		Appropriateness Criteria (Median Score)[a]
	Evaluation of Chest Pain Syndrome	
1.	• Low pretest probability of CAD • EGG interpretable AND able to exercise	I (2.0)
2.	• Low pretest probability of CAD • EGG uninterpretable OR unable to exercise	U (6.5)
3.	• Intermediate pretest probability of CAD • EGG interpretable AND able to exercise	A (7.0)
4.	• Intermediate pretest probability of CAD • ECG uninterpretable OR unable to exercise	A (9.0)
5.	• High pretest probability of CAD • ECG interpretable AND able to exercise	A (8.0)
6.	• High pretest probability of CAD • ECG uninterpretable OR unable to exercise	A (9.0)
	Acute Chest Pain (in Reference to Rest Perfusion Imaging)	
7.	• Intermediate pretest probability of CAD • ECG—no ST elevation AND initial cardiac enzymes negative	A (9.0)
8.	• High pretest probability of CAD • ECG—ST elevation	I (1.0)
	New-Onset/Diagnosed Heart Failure with Chest Pain Syndrome	
9.	• Intermediate pretest probability of CAD	A (8.0)

[a]Median scores of 3.5 and 6.5 are rounded to the middle (uncertain).
Note: I, inappropriate; U, uncertain; A, appropriate.

REFERENCE:

Brindis RG, Douglas PS, Hendel RC, et al. ACCF/ASNC appropriateness criteria for single-photon emission computed tomography myocardial perfusion imaging (SPECT MPI): a report of the American College of Cardiology Foundation Quality Strategic Directions Committee Appropriateness Criteria Working Group and the American Society of Nuclear Cardiology endorsed by the American Heart Association. *J Am Coll Cardiol.* 2005;46(8):1587–1605.

37. ANSWER: C. This is an asymptomatic patient with very low Framingham risk score. Stress SPECT study is considered inappropriate as is a coronary angiogram (Table 3-2.)

TABLE 3-2	Detection of CAD: Asymptomatic (Without Chest Pain Syndrome)	
Indication		Appropriateness Criteria (Median Score)[a]
	Asymptomatic	
10.	• Low coronary heart disease (CHD) risk (Framingham risk criteria)	I (1.0)
11.	• Moderate CHD risk (Framingham)	U (5.5)
	New-Onset or Diagnosed Heart Failure or Left Ventricular Systolic Dysfunction Without Client Pain Syndrome	
12.	• Moderate CHD risk (Framingham)	A (7.5)
	• No prior CAD evaluation AND no planned cardiac catheterization	
	Valvular Heart Disease Without Chest Pain Syndrome	
13.	• Moderate CHD risk (Framingham)	U (5.5)
	• To help guide decision for invasive studies	
	New-Onset Atrial Fibrillation	
14.	• Low CHD risk (Framingham)	U (3.5)
	• Part of the evaluation	
15.	• High CHD risk (Framingham)	A (8.0)
	• Part of the evaluation	
	Ventricular Tachycardia	
16.	• Moderate to high CHD risk (Framingham)	A (9.0)

[a]Median scores of 3.5 and 6.5 are rounded to the middle (uncertain).

Note: I, inappropriate; U, uncertain; A, appropriate.

REFERENCE:

Brindis RG, Douglas PS, Hendel RC, et al. ACCF/ASNC appropriateness criteria for single-photon emission computed tomography myocardial perfusion imaging (SPECT MPI): a report of the American College of Cardiology Foundation Quality Strategic Directions Committee Appropriateness Criteria Working Group and the American Society of Nuclear Cardiology endorsed by the American Heart Association. *J Am Coll Cardiol.* 2005;46(8):1587–1605.

38. ANSWER: B. This is a patient with intermediate-risk score and high-risk occupation. He is able to exercise but has a potentially nondiagnostic baseline ECG. A stress test with an imaging modality is recommended (Table 3-3).

REFERENCE:

Brindis RG, Douglas PS, Hendel RC, et al. ACCF/ASNC appropriateness criteria for single-photon emission computed tomography myocardial perfusion imaging (SPECT MPI): a report of the American College of Cardiology Foundation Quality Strategic Directions Committee Appropriateness Criteria Working Group and the American Society of Nuclear Cardiology endorsed by the American Heart Association. *J Am Coll Cardiol.* 2005;46(8):1587–1605.

TABLE 3-3 Risk Assessment: General and Specific Patient Populations	
Indication	Appropriateness Criteria (Median Score)
Asymptomatic	
17. • Low CHD risk (Framingham)	I (1.0)
18. • Moderate CHD risk (Framingham)	U (4.0)
19. • Moderate to high CHD risk (Framingham) • High-risk occupation (e.g., airline pilot)	A (8.0)
20. • High CHD risk (Framingham)	A (7.5)

Note: I, inappropriate; U, uncertain; A, appropriate.

39. ANSWER: D. This is an asymptomatic patient with a prior normal stress test within 2 years. No further testing is indicated (Table 3-4).

TABLE 3-4 Risk Assessment with Prior Test Results	
Indication	Appropriateness Criteria (Median Score)
Asymptomatic OR Stable Symptoms **Normal Prior SPECT MPI Study**	
21. • Normal initial RNI study • High CHD risk (Framingham) • Annual SPECT MPI study	I (3.0)
22. • Normal initial RNI study • High CHD risk (Framingham) • Repeat SPECT MPI study after 2 years or greater	A (7.0)

REFERENCE:

Brindis RG, Douglas PS, Hendel RC, et al. ACCF/ASNC appropriateness criteria for single-photon emission computed tomography myocardial perfusion imaging (SPECT MPI): a report of the American College of Cardiology Foundation Quality Strategic Directions Committee Appropriateness Criteria Working Group and the American Society of Nuclear Cardiology endorsed by the American Heart Association. *J Am Coll Cardiol.* 2005;46(8):1587–1605.

40. ANSWER: A. This is a low-risk asymptomatic patient undergoing a low-risk surgery. She can exercise >4 METs without difficulty. Preoperative stress testing is not indicated and will not alter her risk or management (Table 3-5).

TABLE 3-5 Risk Assessment: Preoperative Evaluation for Noncardiac Surgery: Intermediate-Risk Surgery	
32. • Minor to intermediate perioperative risk predictor • Normal exercise tolerance (≥4 METS)	I (3.0)

REFERENCE:

Brindis RG, Douglas PS, Hendel RC, et al. ACCF/ASNC appropriateness criteria for single-photon emission computed tomography myocardial perfusion imaging (SPECT MPI): a report of the American College of Cardiology Foundation Quality Strategic Directions Committee Appropriateness Criteria Working Group and the American Society of Nuclear Cardiology endorsed by the American Heart Association. *J Am Coll Cardiol.* 2005;46(8):1587–1605.

41. ANSWER: C. Patients with autonomic dysfunction. The risk of serious hypotension may be higher in patients with autonomic dysfunction, hypovolemia, left main coronary artery stenosis, stenotic valvular heart disease, pericarditis or pericardial effusions, or stenotic carotid artery disease with cerebrovascular insufficiency. Gender and the presence of peripheral vascular disease do not increase the risks of hypotension.

42. ANSWER: B. The most common adverse reactions (≥5%) to regadenoson are dyspnea, headache, flushing, chest discomfort, angina pectoris or ST segment depression, dizziness, chest pain, nausea, abdominal discomfort, dysgeusia, and feeling hot. Most adverse reactions began soon after dosing, and generally resolved within ~15 minutes, except for headache, which resolved in most patients within 30 minutes.

43. ANSWER: C. The interobserver agreement rate was very similar for adenosine–adenosine versus adenosine–regadenoson for three independent blinded readers and varied from 61% to 64%; there were no differences between serial adenosine and adenosine–regadenoson (Fig. 3.1).

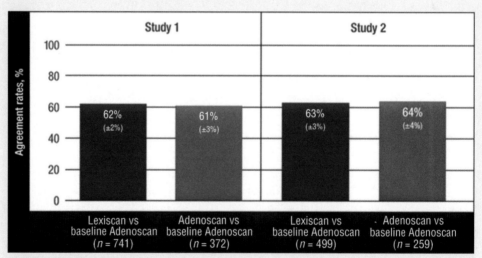

Figure 3.1

REFERENCES:

Iskandrian AE, Bateman TM, Belardinelli L, et al. Adenosine versus regadenoson comparative evaluation in myocardial perfusion imaging: results of the ADVANCE phase 3 multicenter international trial. *J Nucl Cardiol.* 2007;14:645–658.

Lexiscan (regadenoson) injection [package insert]. Deerfield, IL: Astellas Pharma US, Inc.

CHAPTER 4

Imaging Protocols

Manuel D. Cerqueira

QUESTIONS

1. In the simultaneous acquisition dual-isotope protocol, when are the resting thallium-201 images acquired relative to the stress technetium-99m?

   A. Before

   B. At the same time

   C. After

   D. On a separate day

2. What is the most typical image artifact due to patient motion during single photon emission computed tomography (SPECT) acquisition?

   A. Ramp

   B. Hurricane

   C. Ring

   D. Skewed

3. What is the most likely cause of the abnormality noted in the bull's-eye display, Figure 4.1, for a rest/stress rubidium-82 positron emission tomography (PET) perfusion study?

   A. Incorrect definition of the long axis

   B. Incorrect definition of the base slice

   C. Incorrect definition of the apex

   D. Incorrect alignment of the stress/rest

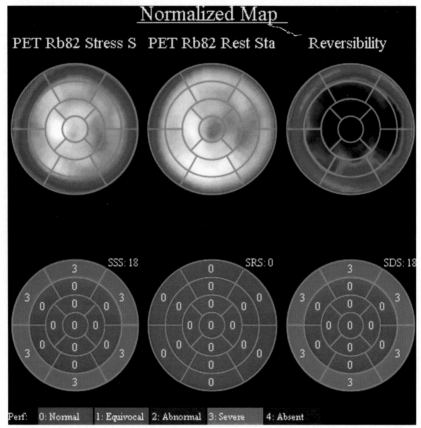

Figure 4.1

4. What is the minimum peak pixel count in the left ventricular (LV) myocardium on a planar technetium-99m SPECT projection that is recommended to obtain best-quality interpretable images?

   A. 50

   B. 100

   C. 150

   D. 200

5. Which of the following parameters will increase the total counts acquired on a SPECT technetium-99m study?

   A. Continuous acquisition

   B. High-resolution collimation

   C. Narrow energy window

   D. Electrocardiogram (ECG) gating

6. Which of the following is most likely to cause transient ischemic dilation (TID) of the left ventricle on SPECT perfusion imaging?

    A. Mild aortic stenosis

    B. Mitral regurgitation

    C. Microvascular coronary disease

    D. Nonischemic cardiomyopathy

7. What is the minimum number of acquisition projections or stops recommended for SPECT acquisition over 180 degrees using technetium-99m radiotracers?

    A. 20

    B. 40

    C. 60

    D. 80

8. What is the best reason to use 16 ECG-gated frames for technetium-99m SPECT acquisition?

    A. Higher counts in each frame

    B. Assessment of diastolic function

    C. Improved perfusion spatial resolution

    D. Better averaging of end systole for more accurate ejection fraction (EF)

9. During filtered back projection reconstruction of SPECT technetium-99m images, what effect does overfiltering have on the perfusion images?

    A. Leaves too much contrast

    B. Leaves too little contrast

    C. Accentuates ramp artifacts

    D. Improves detection of disease

10. What is the mechanism by which prone imaging improves diagnostic accuracy in SPECT perfusion imaging?

    A. Correcting for attenuation

    B. Shifting the location of attenuation

    C. Decreasing patient motion

    D. Shortening imaging time

11. When performing SPECT thallium-201 imaging, how many different energy peaks can be acquired to maximize counts?

    A. 1

    B. 2

    C. 3

    D. 4

12. What is the best explanation for why emission (perfusion) and transmission (computed tomography [CT] for attenuation correction) registration must be verified when using hybrid SPECT/CT and PET/CT systems for rest/stress perfusion imaging?

    A. Patients change beds between emission and transmission acquisition.

    B. Emission and transmission images are acquired simultaneously.

    C. Minor motion and respiratory changes can cause artifacts.

    D. Not necessary but a recommended quality control measure.

13. Which of the following quality control measurements for SPECT systems is required on a daily basis?

    A. Uniformity

    B. Center of rotation

    C. Sensitivity

    D. Resolution and linearity

14. A 69-year-old male has a history of a prior infarction and percutaneous coronary intervention (PCI). He is now having right-sided chest pain and is referred for pharmacologic dual-isotope myocardial perfusion imaging (MPI). Based on Figure 4.2, what is the most likely diagnosis?

    A. Normal study

    B. Lateral wall ischemia and infarction

    C. Septal ischemia

    D. Septal infarction

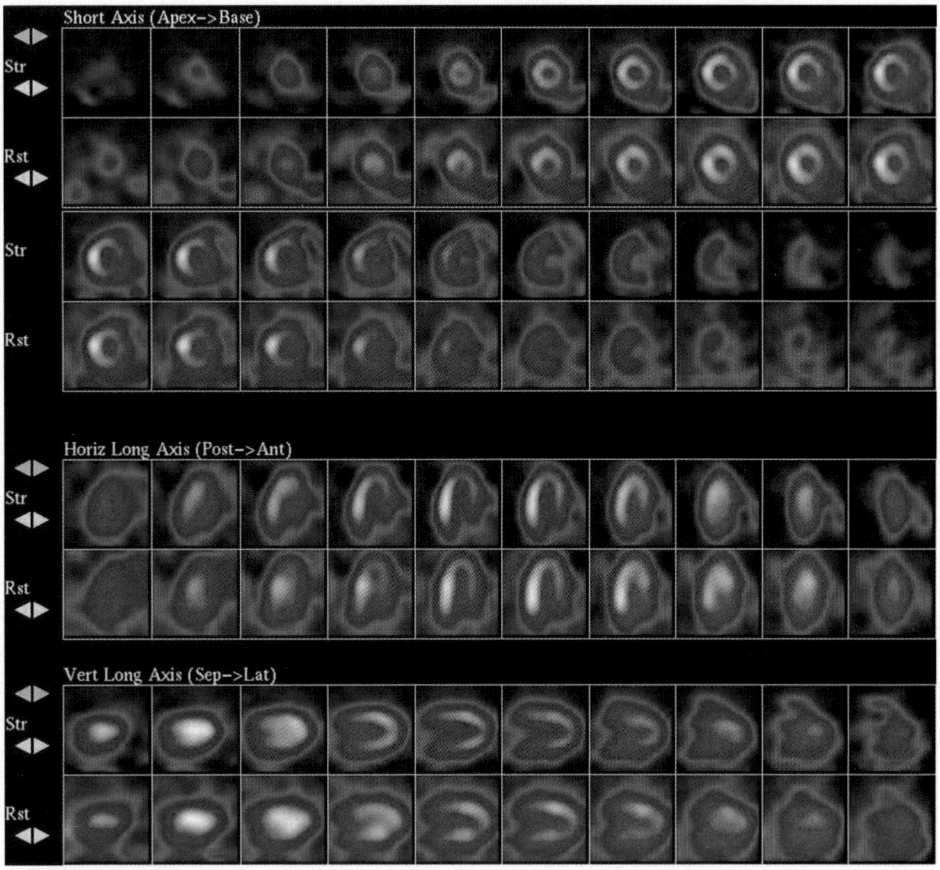

Figure 4.2

15. A 38-year-old male presents with a 1-year history of exertional chest pain that has been increasing in severity over the last week. He is referred for an exercise stress dual-isotope SPECT MPI. During exercise, he develops chest pain. The 3-minute recovery ECG (Fig. 4.3A) and the perfusion images and quantitation (Fig. 4.3B) are shown. What is the next best management option for this patient?

    A. Office visit in 3 weeks

    B. Start aspirin (ASA) and beta-blockers

    C. Elective CT coronary angiography

    D. Hospitalization for coronary angiography

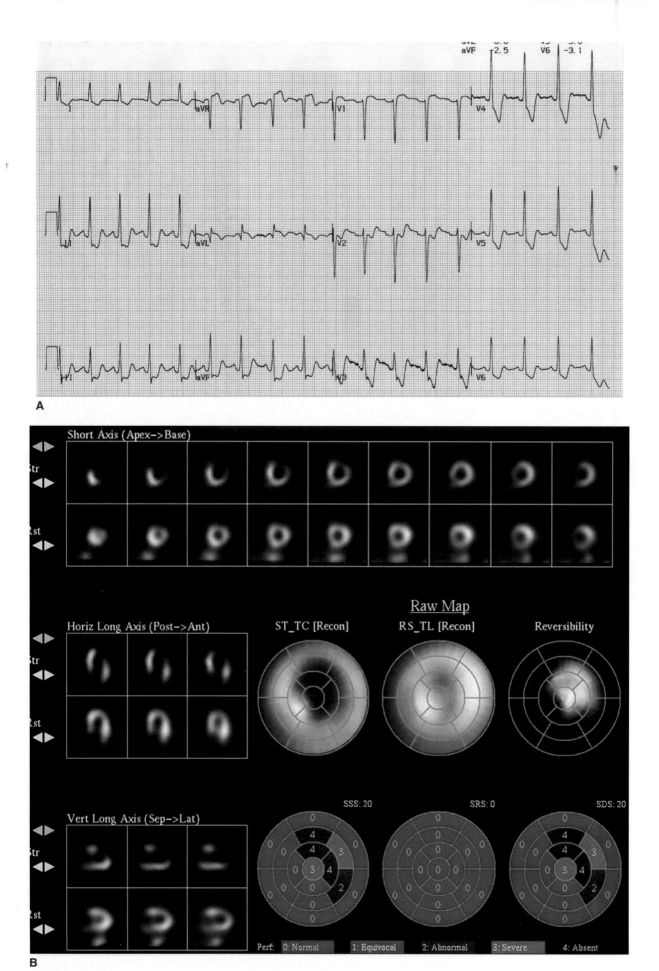

A

B

Figure 4.3A,B

16. A 52-year-old female presented initially with exertional chest pain and shortness of breath (SOB). An exercise stress dual-isotope SPECT MPI was performed (Fig. 4.4A), and the patient was referred for coronary angiography, which showed a tight left anterior descending artery (LAD) lesion treated with PCI. She did well for 3 weeks but developed left jaw discomfort that worsened with exercise at the same time that she had a suspected left mandibular dental abscess. She was referred for a repeat exercise stress SPECT MPI (Fig. 4.4B). Based on these images, what is the next best treatment for this patient?

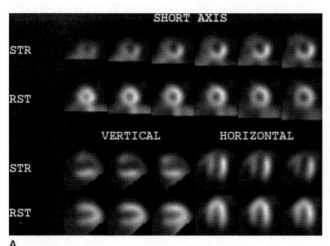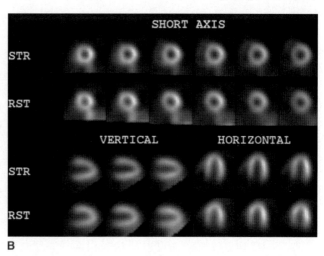

A **B**
Figure 4.4A,B

    A. Refer for coronary angiography.

    B. Immediate hospitalization.

    C. Continue current medical management.

    D. Refer for dental evaluation.

17. A 52-year-old male with a history of a PCI of the right coronary artery 6 months ago is referred for exercise stress dual-isotope SPECT MPI after he develops exertional dyspnea. He exercises to 8 METs, 75% of the maximal age-predicted heart rate without ECG changes but develops SOB and mild chest discomfort. Based on the images shown in Figure 4.5, what is the next best step for management?

    A. Continue current medical management.

    B. Refer for elective pulmonary evaluation.

    C. Refer for dobutamine stress echocardiography.

    D. Hospitalization and urgent coronary angiography.

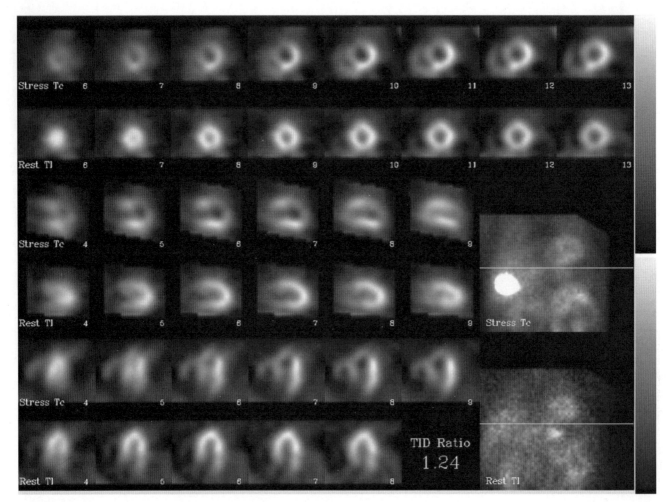

Figure 4.5

ANSWERS

1. ANSWER: B. For the simultaneous acquisition protocol, the resting thallium-201 and stress technetium-99m perfusion images are acquired at the same time. This protocol simplifies acquisition and relies on the use of multiple energy windows to acquire the lower-energy thallium-201 at the same time as the higher-energy technetium-99m. A third window is used to correct for the down scatter of the higher-energy technetium-99m into the lower thallium-201 window. The patient is first injected with thallium-201, usually at the normal dose of 3 to 4 millicuries, and then, stress is performed using a lower dose, 9 to 15 millicuries, of technetium-99m. This allows a single acquisition and saves total protocol time. It is not used widely.

2. ANSWER: B. Patient motion in the vertical, horizontal, or rotational planes causes decreased counts in walls that are contralateral or 180 degrees opposite to each other and usually do not follow coronary artery territory distribution. At the edges of the defects, tails or streaming effects may be noted and are responsible for the "hurricane" appearance, which gives this artifact a name. Motion correction may be used to compensate movement, but it can only correct in the vertical plane. Horizontal and rotational motions are much more difficult to detect on the raw projection images and cannot be corrected.

The ramp filter artifact is seen during filtered back projection using a ramp filter and is caused by overlapping or adjacent liver or bowel activity and causes a loss of counts in the adjacent myocardial walls. The use of iterative reconstruction minimizes this artifact but does not make it go away completely. Waiting longer to get liver clearance or administration of small amounts of liquids to enhance peristalsis and move gastrointestinal activity may allow repeat imaging to improve image quality.

Ring artifacts are seen with nonuniformity across the camera head, which may be due to problems with any of the following: photomultiplier tubes, damaged collimator, camera electronics, or sodium iodide crystal. Daily floods are critical to detecting problems at any of these levels.

Skewed artifacts occur when there are errors in the center of rotation, which cause misregistration during reconstruction and a blurring or skewing of the perfusion data.

3. ANSWER: B. The bull's-eye display (Fig. 4.6) shows severe circumferential reduction in the basal slices for the stress images. There is no combination of coronary lesions that would give this distribution of defects, and this artifact is seen when the base of the left ventricle is incorrectly defined in the lung fields. All the quantitative programs have to deal with hearts of different sizes, and for normal file comparison, hearts have to be expanded or shrunk to a common size. All of the perfusion tracers are taken up by the thick LV walls and there is minimal uptake in normal right ventricles and no uptake in the atria. For that reason, the definition of the basal slices of the left ventricle is critical for accurate quantitative analysis. A first approximation is performed by the computer, but this needs to be visually verified and adjusted.

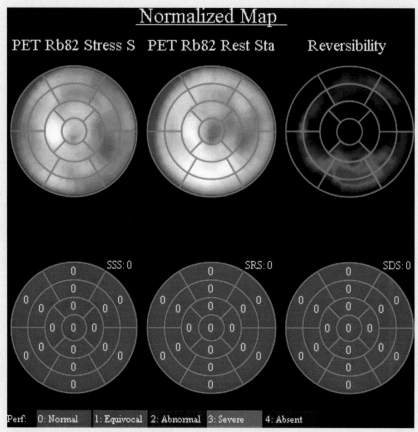

Figure 4.6

When the basal plane is put in the left atrium or lung field, quantitative programs shrink the heart to a common size, and when radiotracer is not detected in the basal slices, it assumes that there is severe ischemia when a comparison to normals is performed. When the basal slices are correctly identified on the stress images (Fig. 4.1), quantitative comparison shows that the study is normal. Careful attention is required to define the basal and apical slices, the long axis of the left ventricle, and coregistration between the stress and rest images in order to obtain accurate quantitative analysis. The insertion of the right ventricle is used to register the "clockwise" rotation of the left ventricle. These rules for quantitation are applicable to both PET and SPECT perfusion imaging and are relatively similar for the major software vendors.

4. ANSWER: D. The greater the number of counts in the myocardium, the higher the quality of the images and the more accurate the interpretation. A minimum of 200 counts/pixel using technetium-99m and 100 counts/pixel using thallium-201 in the myocardium on an anterior projection is recommended. Fewer counts will introduce artifacts due to poor performance of the reconstruction filters, which are usually fixed regardless of the total counts acquired. The total number of counts is influenced by the following: body habitus or body mass index, level of exercise or pharmacologic stress, administered dose of radiopharmaceutical, acquisition time, energy window, and the type of collimator. Dose infiltration at the intravenous insertion site and residual activity in the injection syringe may lower the total dose received by the patient. This means that the delivered dose into the patient is less than the measured dose from the dose calibrator.

REFERENCE:

ASNC Imaging Guidelines and Standards for Single Photon Emission Computed Tomography-2010 http://www.asnc.org/section_73.cfm

5. ANSWER: A. Continuous acquisition allows the gamma camera to acquire counts while it is rotating from one position to the next and increases total counts by eliminating the dead time during camera motion associated with conventional step-and-shoot acquisition. Although there may be image blurring due to the motion, the higher counts and application of appropriate filtering can eliminate the deleterious effects. High-resolution collimation decreases the total counts relative to the use of a general all-purpose collimator. Narrowing the energy window will lower the total counts. ECG gating has minimal effect on counts if separate channels are used to acquire the perfusion data, without applying arrhythmia rejection, and a second channel that acquires the gated information for functional analysis. If only a single channel is used to simultaneously acquire the perfusion and gated information, and arrhythmia rejection is applied, rejected beats will lower the total number of counts in the perfusion images due to beat rejection. This will cause deterioration in the perfusion images, and it is recommended that under these conditions, a very large acceptance window be used to avoid losing counts or prolonging the acquisition if a minimum number of beats or total counts in the myocardium are required.

REFERENCE:

ASNC Imaging Guidelines and Standards for Single Photon Emission Computed Tomography-2010 http://www.asnc.org/section_73.cfm

6. ANSWER: C. Typically transient ischemic dilatation is caused by severe, multivessel proximal epicardial coronary artery disease (CAD) causing subendocardial ischemia that makes the walls of the left ventricle look thinner and the cavity bigger relative to the resting study. Microvascular coronary disease due to hypertension, diabetes, and renal failure may also result in TID. There may be relatively uniform perfusion when scaled or normalized images are visually interpreted despite a marked decrease in absolute blood flow. Measurements of absolute blood flow may be necessary to identify the presence of diffuse disease.

Severe aortic stenosis may cause subendocardial ischemia in the absence of epicardial or microvascular CAD due to an increase in wall tension with exercise or vasodilator stress, which increases resistance in the coronary circulation. This is accentuated by drops in systemic systolic blood pressure, which decreases the driving gradient across the coronary circulation. Mild aortic stenosis should not cause such adverse hemodynamic changes in coronary blood flow. Mitral regurgitation should decrease LV volume due to an increase in regurgitation fraction and an increase in heart rate, which will shorten the diastolic filling period. Nonischemic cardiomyopathies in the absence of CAD should have increased LV volumes at rest and with stress without visually noticeable changes.

7. ANSWER: C. The number of recommended projections is related to the optimal resolution of the imaging system, which includes the radiotracer. Since technetium-99m images provide higher resolution, the minimum number of projections recommended is 60 to 64. For thallium-201 that has lower resolution, 32 projections are acceptable.

8. ANSWER: B. With 16 frames, there is adequate temporal resolution to accurately assess the 4 phases of diastolic filling and measure peak filling rate and the time to peak filling rate. With 8 frames, there is insufficient temporal sampling of diastole to get reliable information.

With 16 frames, the counts in each frame are half of those obtained with 8 frames. The number of frames does not impact on the spatial resolution of the perfusion data if it is acquired with independent channels for gated and nongated data. When using 8 frames, especially at slower heart rates, the poor temporal resolution often does not capture the true end systolic volume and the EF is underestimated relative to when measuring at a higher temporal resolution. It has been shown with equilibrium radionuclide angiography that 50 to 60 ms temporal resolution is required to get accurate EF measurements.

9. ANSWER: B. Overfiltering SPECT perfusion images, which generally have a low signal-to-noise ratio, makes the images too smooth and leaves too little contrast so that there is a loss of information and a tendency to decrease sensitivity for detection of CAD. Typically, Hanning or Butterworth filters are used with filtered back projection and cutoff frequencies are preset and kept constant for all studies to provide a consistency in the images generated. Ideally, the frequency should vary depending on the actual derived signal-to-noise ratio, but this is seldom done in clinical practice. Ramp filter artifacts are caused by the second filter applied during filtered back projection and are less affected by overfiltering. Filters with cutoff frequencies that vary depending on the actual measured signal-to-noise ratio are available but not in wide use.

10. ANSWER: B. Prone imaging was initially used to get greater separation between the inferior wall of the heart and the diaphragm in order to differentiate an inferior wall infarction from the normal loss in counts caused by the diaphragm, which attenuates to a greater extent than the lung tissue that overlaps the majority of the heart. Prone imaging shifts the location of attenuation relative to supine positioning, and the change in attenuation associated with the change in position can be compared. If a defect is caused by attenuation, the location will shift with a shift in body position while a true infarct will be present regardless of patient position. Subsequent studies have demonstrated that prone imaging may also improve identification of both breast and chest wall fat attenuation by observing the shift in attenuation position. Prone imaging does not correct for attenuation as occurs with CT and line source attenuation correction. For obese patients, the prone position may be uncomfortable and result in greater motion, especially when it is performed after supine imaging. Many facilities shorten the prone imaging acquisition to minimize patient discomfort and subsequent motion, but this does not decrease the total imaging time if it is performed in addition to the supine acquisition. Most sites employing prone images do it selectively in problem patients.

11. ANSWER: C. The majority of thallium-201 emission is predominately at the lower 70-keV peak, which is routinely imaged, but there are also peaks at 135 and 167 keV. Newer cameras allow acquisition using several energy windows, and all three peaks should be utilized to increase counts and improve image quality. By increasing counts, the thallium-201 dose administered can be reduced in order to lower total patient radiation exposure.

12. ANSWER: C. Hybrid systems have CT and gamma camera gantries that are contiguous and patients are moved on the table from one system into the other. Bed changes are not required. CT and emission studies are acquired sequentially, not simultaneously, so that there is time and opportunity to shift position between the two studies and even minor motion, such as that due to normal or exaggerated breathing, in any dimension will cause misregistration and inappropriate adding or subtracting of counts during attenuation correction. Such misregistration may create perfusion defects and result in incorrect diagnoses. Verification of accurate emission and transmission registration is both recommended and necessary to assure highest accuracy.

13. ANSWER: A. Uniformity testing and energy peaking are required on a daily basis. Center of rotation is mandatory but varies with the system and is usually not a daily requirement. Some systems have built in verification and correction of center of rotation. Sensitivity testing is an optional measurement. Resolution and linearity are recommended and vary with the manufacturer but neither is required on a daily basis.

14. ANSWER: C. This patient has dextrocardia with situs inversus totalis. On the rotating projection images, not shown, the liver and gallbladder are located on the left side of the abdominal cavity while the heart is on the right side of the chest. From the information provided in the perfusion images alone, the diagnosis can be made as the right ventricle can be seen coming off on the right side in the basal short-axis slices. This is where the lateral wall would normally be seen, which in presence of dextrocardia makes it the septum. This extent of the septal perfusion defect is greater on the stress than on the rest images, which is consistent with ischemia. There is no infarction in the basal septum, but the loss in counts is the normal septal dropout that is observed at the base of the heart. The patient had diagnostic coronary angiography and had septal perforator stenosis. It was not revascularized.

15. ANSWER: D. Despite his young age, the patient had symptoms over 1 year and has a high-risk clinical history due to the increasing symptoms over the week prior to evaluation. The ECG stress test is markedly positive with ST depression and symptoms. The perfusion images show large areas of severe LAD and left circumflex artery distribution ischemia with marked TID of the cavity. This is a high-risk scan with a possible left main distribution and an elective office visit in 3 weeks places this patient at high risk for events. ASA and beta-blockers should be started but that alone is not sufficient with the clinical scenario and the results of stress testing. CT coronary angiography is not indicated based on the high posttest probability of disease and certainly not on an elective basis. Immediate hospitalization with initiation of aggressive medical management and early coronary angiography is the best management option. On coronary angiography, the patient was found to have severe diffuse three-vessel CAD and was referred for coronary artery bypass graft (CABG).

16. ANSWER: D. The initial study (A) shows extensive LAD distribution ischemia that was aggressively treated. When her symptoms returned, there was uncertainty as they were different from her initial symptoms and the presence of a dental cause for the symptoms. The repeat exercise stress SPECT MPI is normal. When SPECT MPI is performed within the first few weeks after PCI, perfusion studies may be positive in the absence of anatomic thrombosis or restenosis. Such perfusion abnormalities have been attributed to endothelial dysfunction and vascular wall instability early after vessel manipulation or the presence of stent coatings that prevent re-endothelialization in the arterial wall. Since this patient study was normal, it is not likely that this patient has mechanical stent malfunction or thrombosis. On the basis of these findings, coronary angiography and immediate hospitalization are not required. Continuing current medical management is important, but on the base of the suspected dental abscess, referral for dental evaluation is needed.

17. ANSWER: D. The images show a high-risk scan with LAD distribution ischemia and TID of the cavity. Although continuing current medical management and referral for pulmonary evaluation are needed, given the severity of the ischemia, more aggressive management is required. Even though the patient did not reach 85% of the target heart, the extensive ischemia at a submaximal workload does not require another noninvasive stress evaluation given the severity of the observed ischemia and the high posttest probability of critical disease. Hospitalization and urgent coronary angiography are the best management option.

Image Interpretation

Manuel D. Cerqueira

CHAPTER 5

QUESTIONS

1. A 62-year-old male presents with increasing shortness of breath and lower extremity edema. A projection image in the left anterior oblique position from the stress portion of a 1-day rest/stress technetium-99m perfusion single photon emission computed tomography myocardial perfusion imaging (SPECT MPI) study is shown in Figure 5.1. Given the available information, what is the most likely cause of the patient's symptoms?

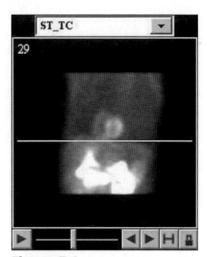

Figure 5.1

A. Pulmonary hypertension

B. Dextrocardia

C. Dilated cardiomyopathy

D. Severe ischemia

2. A patient is referred for a technetium-99m SPECT MPI study. Based on the stress and rest projection images in Figure 5.2, which of the following radio-isotope imaging protocols was most likely used?

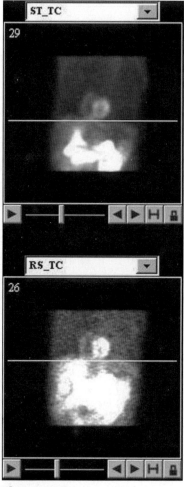

Figure 5.2

A. 1-day stress/rest technetium-99m

B. 1-day rest/stress technetium-99m

C. Rest thallium 201/stress technetium-99m

D. 2-day technetium-99m study

3. Based on the stress and rest projection images shown in Figure 5.3, what is the most likely cause for the patient's severe shortness of breath?

A. Chronic obstructive pulmonary disease (COPD)

B. Dilated cardiomyopathy

C. Hypertrophic cardiomyopathy

D. Pulmonary stenosis

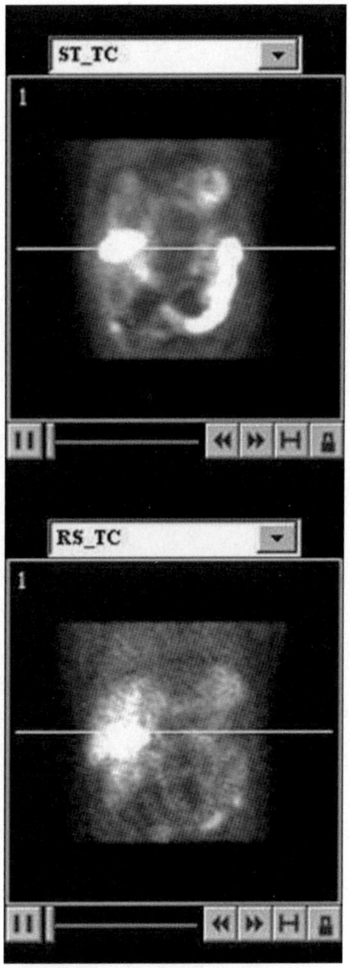

Figure 5.3

4. A 67-year-old male presents with atypical chest pain and an abnormal baseline electrocardiogram (ECG). Serial perfusion images from an exercise stress SPECT MPI at 13.5 METs without anginal symptoms are shown in Figure 5.4. Based on the images, what is the most likely explanation for the findings?

    A. Three-vessel coronary artery disease (CAD)

    B. Scaling artifact

    C. Breast attenuation

    D. Ramp filter artifact

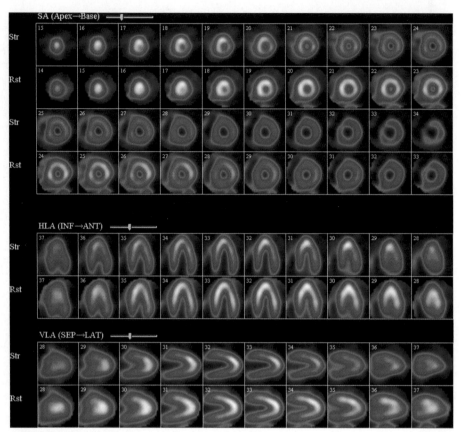

Figure 5.4

5. A 60-year-old female presents with chest pain to the emergency department and is referred for exercise SPECT MPI. Based on Figure 5.5, what is the next best step for management?

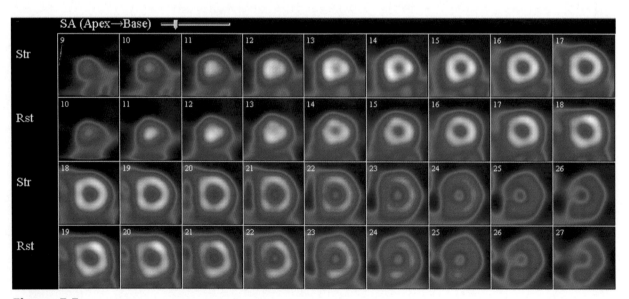

Figure 5.5

A. Coronary angiography

B. Computed tomography (CT) coronary angiography

C. Hospital admission

D. Discharge for outpatient follow-up

6. A 58-year-old female with progressive chest pain is referred for an outpatient stress myocardial perfusion imaging (MPI). Based on Figure 5.6, what is the next best step for this patient?

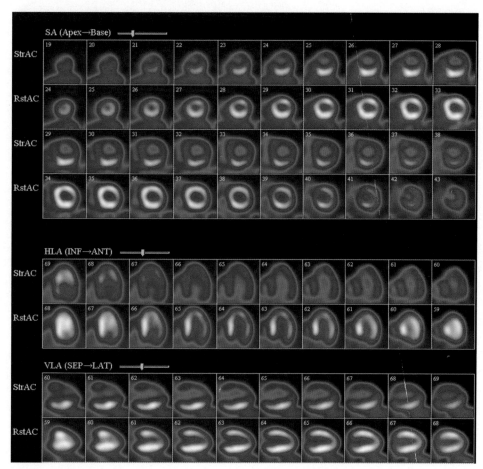

Figure 5.6

A. Aggressive medical therapy

B. Echocardiography

C. CT coronary angiography

D. Coronary angiography

7. A 75-year-old male with a remote myocardial infarction and atypical chest pain is referred for a rubidium-82 vasodilator positron emission tomography (PET) study. The stress and rest images in Figure 5.7 show:

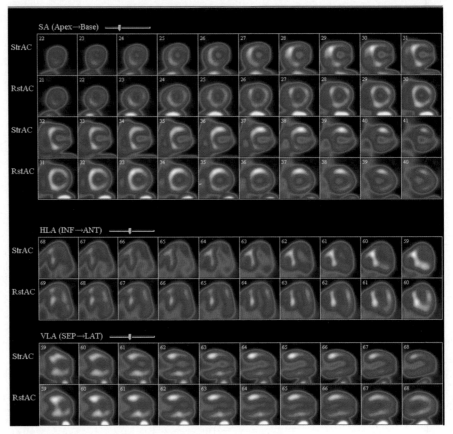

Figure 5.7

   A. Misregistration artifact on the rest images.

   B. Severe lateral wall ischemia.

   C. Severe lateral wall ischemia and apical infarction.

   D. Reconstruction artifact due to gastric uptake.

8. An 85-year-old male with moderate CAD documented 6 years ago presents with atypical chest pain. An exercise stress SPECT MPI is performed and the short-axis view is shown in Figure 5.8. Which coronary artery is likely to be causing the symptoms?

   A. Left anterior descending

   B. Left circumflex

   C. Right coronary artery

   D. Ramus branch

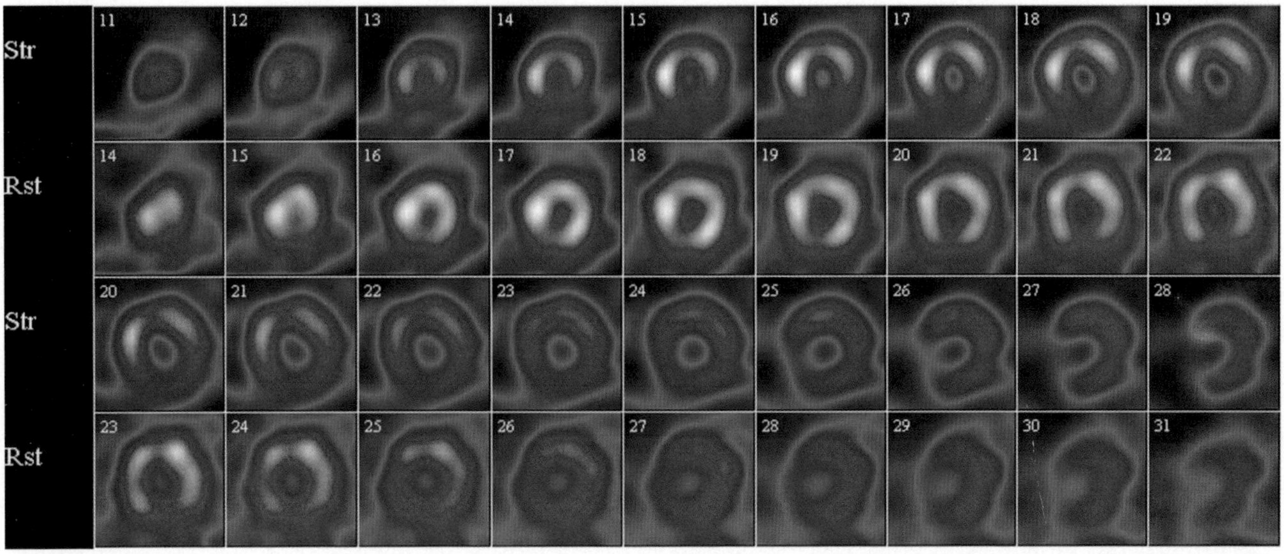

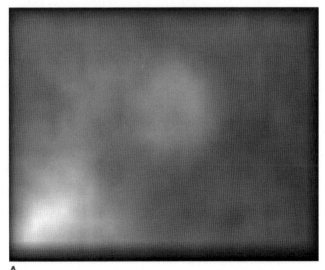

Figure 5.8

9. A 39-year-old female with a body mass index of 45 is being evaluated for intestinal bypass surgery. She has hypertension, diabetes, and markedly elevated cholesterol values. A pharmacologic stress SPECT MPI without attenuation correction is performed. The patient has severe chest pain during pharmacologic stress but no ECG changes. The perfusion study is interpreted as normal. Due to the chest pain symptoms with vasodilator stress, the referring physician is skeptical of the results and wants an explanation. Based on the raw projection image shown in Figure 5.9A, 15th of 64, and short-axis views, Figure 5.9B, what is the most likely explanation for the interpretation?

A
Figure 5.9A

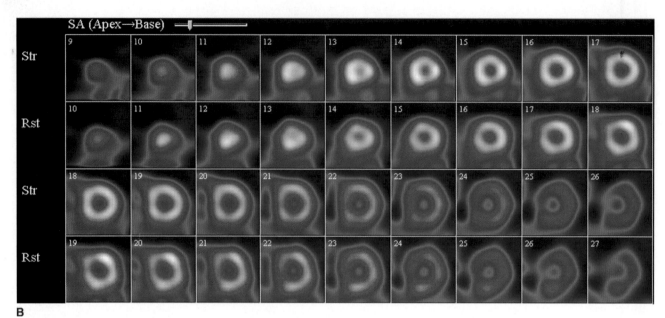

B

Figure 5.9B

A. False-negative study in a high-risk patient

B. Uniform breast attenuation

C. Balanced breast and diaphragmatic attenuation

D. Inconclusive study and further testing required

10. A 24-year-old male develops sharp sternal discomfort after heavy physical exercise. He is referred for an exercise stress SPECT MPI. He exercises for 15 minutes on the Bruce protocol without chest pain or ECG changes of ischemia. During image acquisition, the patient moved (top row of images) and these were motion corrected (second row) and compared to the rest images (Fig. 5.10). Based on the perfusion images shown, what is the optimal next step for this patient's management?

A. Assess cardiovascular risk factors.

B. Measure coronary artery calcium.

C. Refer for coronary angiography.

D. Send for cardiac surgery consultation.

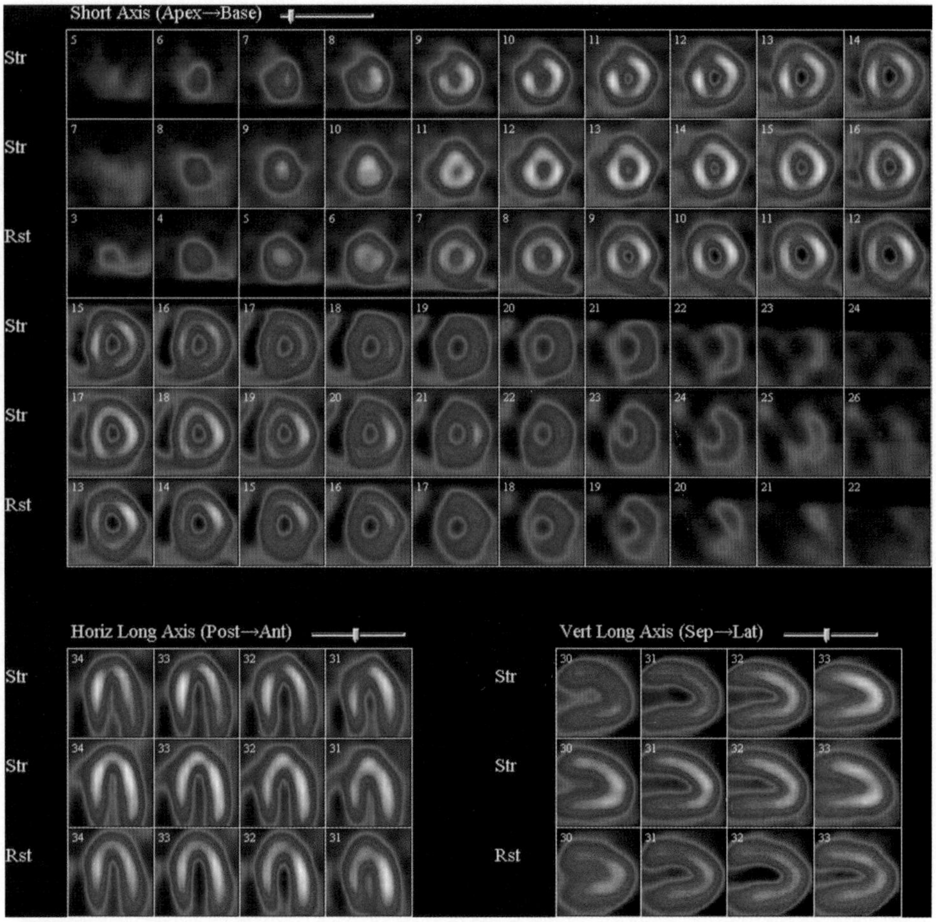

Figure 5.10

11. An 85-year-old female with multiple prior infarctions and a coronary artery bypass graft (CABG) has worsening heart failure symptoms despite optimal medical management. She is referred for an SPECT MPI. Based on Figure 5.11, what is the best next method of management?

    A. Continue medical management

    B. PET assessment of hibernation

    C. CT coronary angiography

    D. Coronary angiography

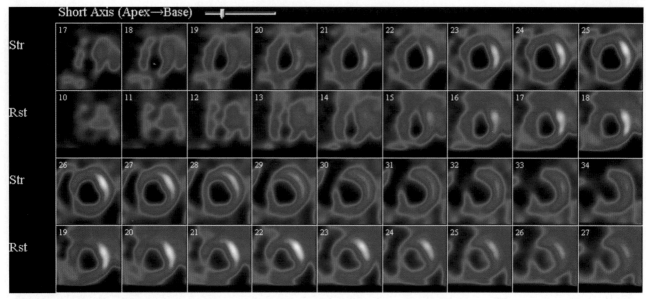

Figure 5.11

12. A 46-year-old female is being evaluated for preoperative risk assessment. She is 5-feet 8-inch tall and weighs 434 pounds. She has diabetes, hypertension, and elevated lipids. She is referred for a pharmacologic 1-day rest/stress technetium-99m perfusion study without (A) and with CT attenuation correction (B). Based on Figure 5.12, what is the correct diagnosis?

   A. Normal study

   B. Inferior infarction

   C. Apical infarction

   D. Nondiagnostic

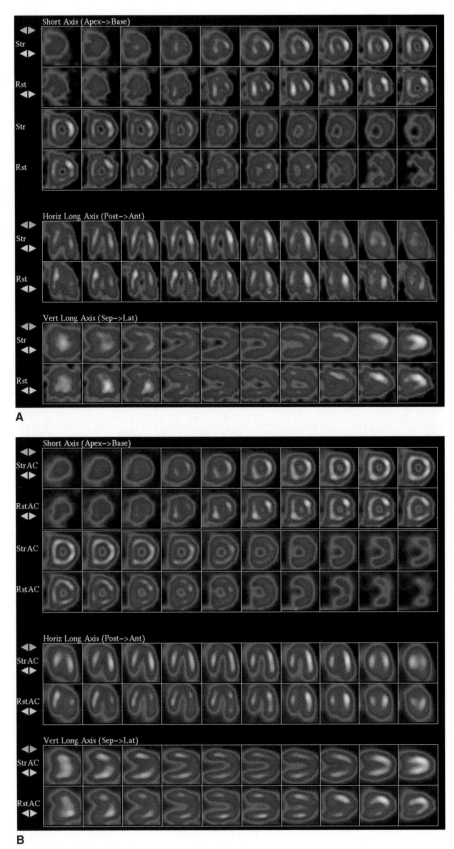

Figure 5.12A,B

ANSWERS ·

1. ANSWER: A. The image shows marked right ventricular hypertrophy and enlargement that is most consistent with pulmonary hypertension due to any cause. The relative paucity of lung uptake of the technetium-99m agent suggests possible obstructive airway disease, which is a frequent cause of pulmonary hypertension and right ventricular hypertrophy. The heart and abdominal organs are in the correct anatomical position, which excludes dextrocardia. Since the left ventricle is normal in size, there is no reason to suspect a dilated cardiomyopathy. Although severe ischemia cannot be excluded based on the projection images alone, it is a less likely diagnosis given the available information. When using thallium-201 with stress, there may be increased lung uptake of thallium-201 on the stress images due to severe ischemia, which causes an increase in the lung-to-heart ratio. This is due to a transient elevation of the pulmonary capillary wedge pressure in association with ischemia and the extravasation of thallium-201 from the intravascular into the interstitial space. Such abnormal heart-to-lung ratios in association with serve ischemia have not been reported with technetium-99m agents and ratios are not routinely measured.

2. ANSWER: B. Based on the grainy quality of the rest images due to the low count statistics, we are led to conclude that this is a 1-day study using a low-dose rest, 8 to 12 millicuries, and a high-dose stress, 20 to 30 millicuries, study. In a dual-isotope protocol, the resting thallium-201 images may have a similar granularity due to low counts associated with the lower dose, 2.5 to 4 millicuries, that is administered to avoid high radiation exposure and the slower radioactive decay. We know both agents are technetium-99m based on the biodistribution that includes large amounts of radioactivity in the liver and gastrointestinal (GI) track. Thallium-201 may have some GI uptake but not the high quantity and the linear/tubular pattern that is shown here. This excludes dual-isotope protocol and is most consistent with a low-dose rest/ high-dose stress sequence. A 2-day technetium-99m study could theoretically be done using low-dose rest and high-dose stress as shown, but generally, such studies are performed on heavy patients using high and comparable doses to allow high and comparable doses for both the stress and rest in order to achieve optimal image quality.

3. ANSWER: A. On the rest, but most prominently on the high-dose stress anterior images, there is marked thickening of the diaphragm recognized as a lucency starting from the patient's right abdominal wall and extending all the way to the heart. Both attenuation by the diaphragm muscle and the contrast between the vascular lungs above and the liver-associated technetium-99m uptake give the dark appearance. With severe COPD, there is marked hypertrophy of the diaphragm resulting in such an appearance on the projection images. On the perfusion images, the hypertrophy of the diaphragm causes marked inferior wall attenuation. On these anterior images, the left ventricle is not dilated and a cardiomyopathy is not a likely cause. Heart size can be compared to the thoracic and the cardiothoracic ratio should be <½. Hypertrophic cardiomyopathy cannot be definitively excluded, but it does not generally cause diaphragmatic hypertrophy. Pulmonary stenosis does not cause pulmonary congestion. Ascites and pulmonary effusions may give a similar appearance on the projection images, but these are not options provided.

4. ANSWER: B. The images show a very hot apical anterior hot spot on the stress images (*arrow*) that is causing a scaling artifact. This can be recognized by the circumferential decrease in counts that is most prominent on the short-axis slices relative to the resting images. The incorrect scaling decreases the subendocardial counts and may give the appearance of transient ischemic dilation. Three-vessel CAD is unlikely in view of the high workload, absence of symptoms, and the nonanatomic distribution of the perfusion defects. There is no possible combination of anatomic coronary stenosis that would give such diffuse circumferential decrease in midcavity and basal perfusion without involving the apex.

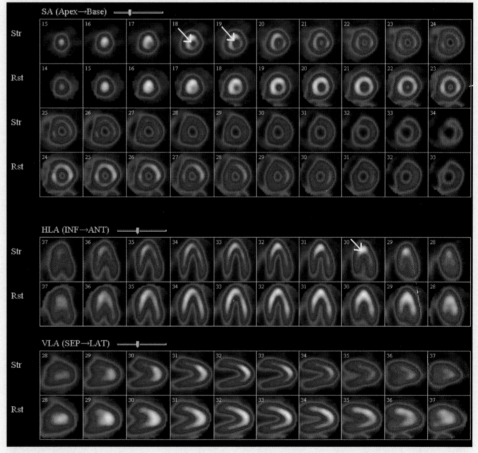

Figure 5.13

Breast attenuation is less common in a male and the diffuse pattern of decreased perfusion is not typical. A ramp filter artifact is caused by a hot loop of bowel or liver adjacent to the heart that results in decreased counts in the nearby wall when using filtered back projection for reconstruction. There is no liver or bowel visualized on the images shown.

5. ANSWER: D. This is a completely normal study by visual and quantitative analysis. The stress images have focal hot spots in the septum and lateral wall near the apex. The bull's-eye display shows completely normal perfusion on the stress and rest images (Fig. 5.14). The normal perfusion makes coronary angiography, CT coronary angiography, and hospital admission unnecessary, and discharge is the best option for this patient.

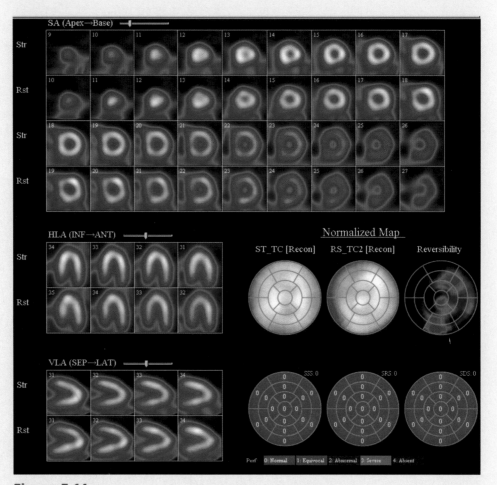

Figure 5.14

6. ANSWER: D. The images demonstrate a large area of severe ischemia involving the apex, septum, anterior, and the lateral walls. There is transient ischemic dilation of the cavity. This is a high-risk scan consistent with severe tight proximal disease in the left anterior descending or left main or diffuse severe multivessel disease. In view of the progressive symptoms, coronary angiography is the best management option. Aggressive medial therapy is indicated but not the best option given the severity of the ischemia. An echocardiogram is of no value in this situation. Given the physiologic demonstration of severe ischemia by SPECT, the patient is likely to benefit from and require revascularization. CT coronary angiography is capable of demonstrating CAD but since revascularization is likely, coronary angiography is the best option as percutaneous coronary intervention (PCI) can be performed during the same session.

7. ANSWER: C. The rubidium-82 images show a large area of severe lateral wall ischemia extending from the apex to the base. There is an apical infarction most prominent on the horizontal and vertical long-axis images.

Misregistration between the attenuation map and perfusion images causes defects due to inappropriate attenuation correction. Since the resting images are normal other than the apical infarction, misregistration is unlikely. Misregistration may be verified by checking the alignment between the image sets and should be done routinely as part of PET study interpretation whether using germanium or CT methods of attenuation correction. Although there is not enough information provided to definitely exclude this option, it is not the best answer. There is definitely lateral wall ischemia, but there is also an apical infarction. PET perfusion images are generally reconstructed using iterative reconstruction that tends to minimize the liver and GI artifacts associated with filtered back projection. Such artifacts are created in the walls adjacent to the hot areas, and in this case, the inferior wall is completely normal, which excludes this as an option.

8. ANSWER: C. The images show a moderately severe perfusion defect in the inferior wall starting at the apex and going all the way to the base. At the midcavity and base, it extends into the contiguous inferolateral wall. This is most consistent with right coronary artery stenosis. The severity and extent is

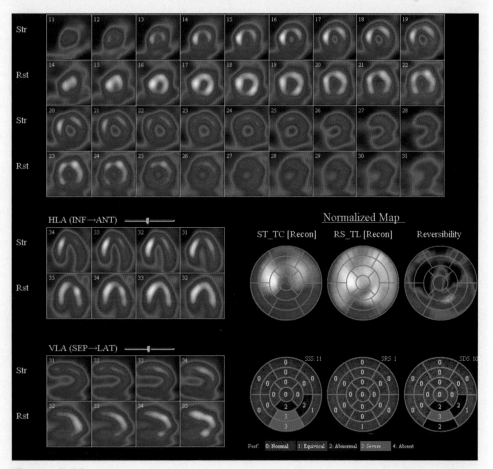

Figure 5.15

best appreciated on the 17-segment bull's-eye display and can be seen in the vertical long-axis images (Fig. 5.15). Inferior and lateral wall defects seen on the short-axis view are best corroborated on the vertical long-axis views. On the horizontal long-axis view, inferior and anterior wall defects are not well appreciated due to minor misregistration in the transaction from the lung, through the myocardium and into the left ventricular cavity. Similarly, defects in the septum and lateral walls in the short-axis views are best corroborated on the horizontal long-axis views.

Although there is great variability in coronary artery topography, a high-grade stenosis in the left anterior, left circumflex, and ramus branch coronary arteries will not give defects in the myocardial segments shown in the perfusion images.

9. ANSWER: B. These images were acquired with a small field of view camera with the patient sitting upright in a chair with the chest pressed against a stabilizing bar. The raw projection image shows a large left breast covering the entire heart. This results in uniform attenuation of the heart and not the focal decrease on the perfusion images usually seen in the anterior wall when there is only partial coverage of the heart by breast tissue. The right breast can be seen on the right and the bright area between is due to underlying liver and lung background that has less attenuation. These rotating projection images should be reviewed in cine mode on a workstation as part of quality control for every study interpreted.

Despite the multiple risk factors usually associated with obesity, the patient's gender and young age put her into a lower-risk category for CAD. Chest pain with vasodilator stress in the absence of CAD is a common finding especially in the absence of ECG changes. In such a clinical situation, SPECT MPI is more likely to have false-positive findings, and false negatives are a less of an occurrence. For these reasons, it is not likely that this is a false-negative study.

Balanced breast and diaphragmatic attenuation is possible when there is only partial covering of the anterior wall by breast tissue and the inferior wall is covered by the diaphragm. The obvious and complete covering of the heart by the left breast as shown makes this an incorrect answer.

With a normal study and clear visualization of the overlying breast tissue, there is confidence in the interpretation and the study is not inconclusive and further testing is not required.

10. ANSWER: A. Based on appropriate use criteria, this patient does not need an SPECT MPI study. The stress images with motion show an anteroseptal defect at the right ventricular insertion site or the left anterior descending grove that is likely an artifact as it improves with motion correction. Given the location, the patient's low pretest risk and the very high exercise capacity in the absence of chest pain or ECG changes, this study should be read as normal. Assessing risk factors is the most conservative and appropriate approach in this clinical situation. The benefit of coronary artery calcium scoring in this situation has no proven value once the results of the stress test are known. Coronary angiography and surgical evaluation are invasive and not indicated.

11. ANSWER: B. These images show extensive and severe areas of absent perfusion on the resting SPECT MPI involving the left anterior descending and right coronary artery territories with only the lateral wall showing perfusion. There is no evidence of ischemia. With this extensive amount of resting perfusion and the patient already on optimal medical management, PET assessment of viability using FDG imaging is a more sensitive test for identifying areas of the myocardium that may be hibernating and capable of regaining mechanical function if they can be successfully revascularized. With this extensive amount of infarction and a probable high calcium score, CT coronary angiography will not be useful. Coronary angiography in the absence of demonstration of hibernation is not likely to lead to a change in management and will not provide additive information.

12. ANSWER: A. The uncorrected images (A) show a fixed inferior wall and apical defect. On the CT attenuation correction images, the inferior wall defect is not present, but there is still apical thinning. These changes are most consistent with a normal study in a challenging patient due to the large body mass index. Typically in an obese female patient, there is partial covering of the anterior wall of the heart by breast tissue, which causes an anterior perfusion defect. In this patient, the breast was so large that it covered the entire heart giving a relatively uniform attenuation. The diaphragm however was elevated due to the increased abdominal pressure caused by the weight of the breasts and abdominal fat causing a severe wall defect. On the gated images, it had normal motion suggesting it was attenuation. With CT attenuation correction (B), the inferior wall was corrected due to the marked attenuation. The apical thinning is still present, and there was normal motion on the gated study suggesting it was apical thinning—a recognized variant. Typically with attenuation correction, the apex usually appears much thinner as the overrepresentation of counts due to close proximity throughout the 180-degree acquisition is corrected.

Cardiovascular Positron Emission Tomography (PET)

Richard C. Brunken

QUESTIONS

1. Which of the following statements best characterizes rubidium-82, a radiotracer frequently used for cardiac PET imaging?

    A. The tracer is eluted from a portable generator, in which decay of the "parent" isotope molybdenum-99 yields the "daughter" isotope rubidium-82.

    B. Following intravenous (IV) administration, rubidium-82 is retained in the myocardium by mitochondrial sequestration.

    C. As part of the quality control (QC) process, the first sample of the day eluted from the rubidium-82 generator is examined for "break-through" of radionuclide contaminants.

    D. The 2-minute half-life of rubidium-82 facilitates patient throughput in busy imaging centers, permitting rest and stress PET myocardial perfusion imaging in as little as 30 minutes.

2. Which of the following PET tracers can be used to quantitatively assess both myocardial perfusion and metabolism?

    A. ^{18}F-2-fluoro-2-deoxy-2-D-glucose (FDG)

    B. ^{11}C-acetate

    C. ^{11}C-heptagluconate

    D. ^{11}C-hydroxyephedrine

3. At a myocardial blood flow of 3.7 mL/min/g tissue, which of the following myocardial perfusion tracers would exhibit the highest net tissue uptake (flow × extraction)?

    A. Thallium-201 chloride

    B. Nitrogen-13 ammonia

    C. Technetium-99m sestamibi

    D. Oxygen-15 water

4. A 64-year-old patient with congestive heart failure and malignant ventricular arrhythmias undergoes cardiac PET imaging with rubidium-82 at rest (RstAC) and ^{18}F-2-fluoro-2-deoxy-2-D-glucose (FDGAC). The FDG images were acquired following oral glucose loading. Representative cardiac PET images are shown in Figure 6.1. Which of the following findings would be most likely to be identified in the *abnormal* anteroapical and basal inferior myocardial regions with the matching defects in perfusion and metabolism on the PET images?

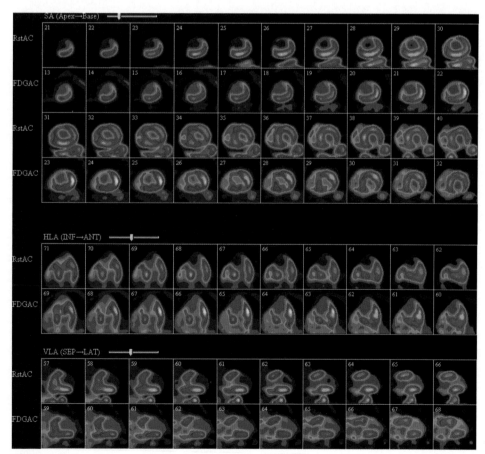

Figure 6.1

A. An increase in signal intensity on delayed gadolinium-enhanced magnetic resonance images

B. An improvement in regional wall motion on a postpremature ventricular contraction on contrast left ventriculography

C. Thallium-201 redistribution on rest and 4-hour redistribution single photon emission computed tomography myocardial perfusion imaging (SPECT MPI)

D. An end-diastolic wall thickness of 8.0 to 8.5 mm on electrocardiogram-gated magnetic resonance images

5. Which of the following myocardial perfusion imaging protocols will deliver the highest effective dose of ionizing radiation to an adult patient?

A. Stress and 4-hour redistribution thallium-201 SPECT imaging (3.5 mCi of thallium-201 chloride)

B. 1-day rest/stress technetium-99m SPECT tetrofosmin imaging (10.0 mCi rest dose, 27.5 mCi stress dose)

C. 2-day rest/stress technetium-99m tetrofosmin SPECT imaging (25.0 mCi rest dose, 25.0 mCi stress dose)

D. Rest and stress rubidium-82 PET imaging (50 mCi rest dose, 50 mCi stress dose)

6. A 59-year-old man is concerned about the possibility of coronary artery disease (CAD). His 64-year-old brother recently sustained a myocardial infarction, and an evaluation performed by his family physician indicates an intermediate probability for CAD. His family physician orders a computed tomography (CT) scan for coronary calcium scoring, and the coronary calcium score is 612. If the patient is referred for an adenosine rubidium-82 PET myocardial perfusion study, which of the following statements would best describe the relationship between the CT findings and the anticipated results of the PET study?

A. The likelihood that the PET study will show ischemia is <2%.

B. The probability that the PET study will demonstrate ischemia is between 25% and 50%.

C. The likelihood that the PET study will demonstrate ischemia exceeds 50%.

D. Once the patient's conventional cardiovascular risk factors are considered, the calcium score provides no incremental benefit for predicting the presence of inducible ischemia on the PET study.

7. The 59-year-old man from the previous question undergoes an adenosine rubidium-82 cardiac PET imaging study. The study is normal, without a reversible perfusion defect to suggest ischemia. Which of the following best describes the patient's annual risk for death/myocardial infarction?

    A. 0.2%

    B. 1%

    C. 5%

    D. 8%

8. A 59-year-old man with atypical chest pain is referred for PET imaging 3 weeks after a stent to the left anterior descending (LAD) artery. He has a history of mixed hyperlipidemia, type II diabetes, hypothyroidism, and adrenal cortical insufficiency. Dipyridamole stress (StrAC) and rest (RstAC) rubidium-82 PET images are shown in Figure 6.2. Which of the following best describes the findings on the PET imaging study?

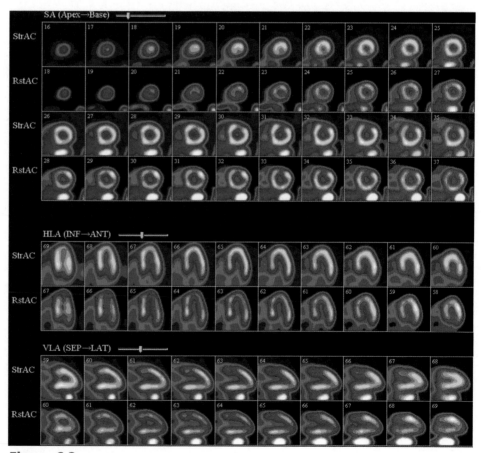

Figure 6.2

    A. Normal study

    B. Reversible defect, mid and distal LAD distribution

    C. Fixed defect, distal LAD distribution

    D. Fixed perfusion defect in a diagonal distribution

9. PET imaging can be performed in a two-dimensional (2D) mode or in a three-dimensional (3D) mode. Which of the following statements best describes the use of 2D versus 3D PET imaging?

    A. In the 2D mode, there are lead or tungsten septa between the detector rings.

    B. As compared with doses used for imaging in the 2D mode, the doses employed for PET imaging in the 3D mode generally need to be larger.

    C. The 2D mode is the type used most frequently for PET oncology imaging.

    D. The 2D mode is preferred when PET imaging is performed in children.

10. Which of the following crystal types used in PET scanners has the highest stopping power for annihilation photons?

    A. Bismuth germanate (BGO)

    B. Lutetium oxyorthosilicate (LSO)

    C. Gadolinium oxyorthosilicate (GSO)

    D. Lutetium yttrium orthosilicate (LYSO)

11. Which of the following types of stress is an indicator of coronary artery endothelial function when used in conjunction with PET myocardial perfusion imaging?

    A. IV dipyridamole

    B. IV adenosine

    C. cold pressor test

    D. IV regadenoson

12. Which of the following QC measures would not be appropriate for a PET/CT scanner?

    A. Center of rotation

    B. System sensitivity

    C. Intrinsic scatter fraction

    D. Accuracy of attenuation correction

13. In which of the following patients might an artifact be observed on myocardial PET images if x-ray CT is used for attenuation correction?

    A. A 56-year-old woman with bilateral silicone breast implants

    B. A 72-year-old man with a permanent pacemaker with RA and RV leads

    C. A 39-year-old woman with cardiac sarcoidosis, ventricular arrhythmias, and an implanted defibrillator with an RV lead

    D. An 82-year-old man with hypertensive heart disease and pronounced mitral annular calcification

14. For which of the following positron-emitting isotopes is the energy of the annihilation photons the greatest?

    A. Fluorine-18

    B. Rubidium-82

    C. Nitrogen-13

    D. Same for each isotope

15. ^{18}F-2-fluoro-2-deoxy-D-glucose, or FDG, is frequently used in clinical PET imaging to assess myocardial viability. In considering dosimetry, which organ receives the highest dose of radiation?

    A. Gallbladder

    B. Myocardium

    C. Urinary bladder

    D. Colon

16. In PET imaging, the term "time of flight" refers to:

   A. The length of time from positron emission by the atomic nucleus to annihilation with an electron.

   B. The period of time that the electron and positron interact with each other prior to their mutual annihilation (i.e., the period of time of existence of "positronium").

   C. The shortest period of time in which a PET detector can distinguish between two independently occurring scintillation events.

   D. The time difference between two annihilation photons reaching their corresponding detectors.

17. Which organ receives the highest radiation dose in a rubidium-82 PET perfusion study?

   A. Kidneys

   B. Gastrointestinal (GI) tract

   C. Urinary bladder

   D. Heart

18. There is increasing public concern regarding the biologic effects of ionizing radiation in medicine. With regard to the biologic effects of ionizing radiation, the term "radiation hormesis" refers to:

   A. A deterministic effect of exposure to ionizing radiation.

   B. A stochastic effect of exposure to ionizing radiation.

   C. A protective effect of exposure to low amounts of ionizing radiation.

   D. The minimal dose of ionizing radiation required to exert a biologic effect.

19. FDG PET/CT imaging is sometimes used to visualize vulnerable plaques in the arterial system. Which of the following methods should be used to acquire the highest-quality images of a coronary arterial plaque?

   A. Using an insulin clamp technique

   B. Using a glucose clamp technique

   C. Following a low-carbohydrate, high-fat meal

   D. Following oral glucose loading

20. Which of the following statements best characterizes the use of FDG PET imaging for visualizing atherosclerotic plaque inflammation?

A. Up-regulation of glucose-6-phosphatase within activated plaque macrophages increases the metabolic trapping of FDG within the arterial plaque.

B. Activated macrophages exhibit an up-regulation of hexokinase, increasing the metabolic trapping of FDG within the plaque.

C. Relative hypoxia in the center of a plaque will impair the metabolic trapping of FDG.

D. Activated macrophages up-regulate GLUT4 transporter levels in the cell membrane, enhancing the metabolic trapping of FDG within the arterial plaque.

21. Which of the following statements correctly identifies the approach for imaging of unstable plaques with FDG PET?

A. PET imaging should begin approximately 45 minutes following tracer injection.

B. PET imaging should begin approximately 1 hour following tracer administration.

C. PET imaging should begin about 2 hours following tracer injection.

D. PET characterization of atherosclerotic plaques is largely unaffected by the time interval from tracer injection to the start of imaging.

22. Stress/rest rubidium-82 perfusion images and FDG metabolic images in a patient with congestive heart failure are shown in Figure 6.3. The study was requested to determine the need for coronary angiography in this patient. Which of the following is shown?

A. Extensive ischemia involving the left anterior, circumflex, and right coronary distributions, with a scar in the right coronary distribution

B. An image display scaling artifact, due to the relatively high degree of GI activity on the rest perfusion images

C. Extensive myocardial hibernation involving the left anterior, circumflex, and right coronary distributions and scar involving the right coronary distribution

D. Extensive myocardial scar involving the left anterior, circumflex, and right coronary distributions and a small area of myocardial hibernation involving the right coronary distribution

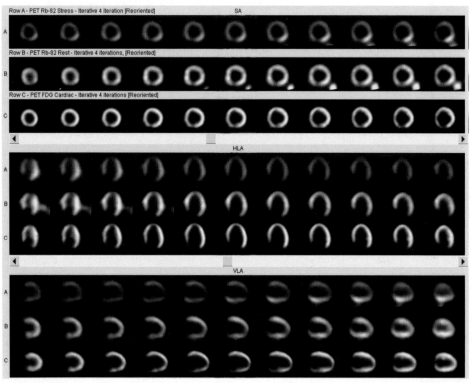

Figure 6.3

23. What is the best explanation in the above case for the left ventricular myocardium appearing thinner and "sharper" on the FDG images compared to the rubidium-82 images?

    A. A greater number of image counts on the FDG study

    B. An artifact of scaling, due to the GI activity adjacent to the heart on the rubidium-82 images

    C. Misalignment of the rubidium-82 emission images and the CT transmission images

    D. The average kinetic energy of the rubidium-82 positron is greater than that of the fluorine-18 positron

24. A nondiabetic patient referred for PET imaging in Los Angeles, California, has a blood glucose level of 79 mg/dL. Which of the following procedures would *not* be appropriate to use as part of a protocol designed to assess myocardial viability with FDG imaging?

    A. Acipimox, 250 mg orally prior to FDG injection

    B. Oral glucose loading with 50 g of dextrose prior to FDG injection

    C. IV glucose loading with D50W to which 20 mg of hydrocortisone has been added to administer a total of 25 g dextrose

    D. "Priming" the patient with 50 mL of 20% dextrose and 5 units of regular insulin IV

25. Nitrogen-13 ammonia and rubidium-82 images from a 69-year-old woman with chest pain are shown in Figure 6.4. The two sets of images were obtained on separate days, and there was no intervening clinical event. Review of the transmission and emission images for both the rubidium-82 and nitrogen-13 studies revealed appropriate alignment. On quantitation of myocardial blood flow on the nitrogen-13 images, rest and stress blood flow measurements were comparable in all myocardial segments, and the calculated flow reserves were 3.9 to 4.0 in all segments. Which of the following best explains the differences in tracer uptake in the inferolateral region of the left ventricle for the two radiotracers?

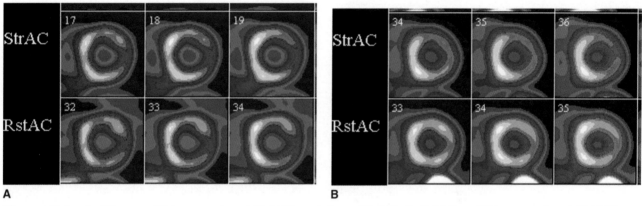

Figure 6.4 **A:** Nitrogen-13 images at rest (RstAC) and stress (StrAC). **B:** Rubidium-82 images at rest (RstAC) and stress (StrAC).

    A. Vasospasm of a marginal vessel at the time of nitrogen-13 ammonia PET imaging

    B. Normal variant of myocardial uptake of nitrogen-13 ammonia

    C. Scaling artifact from liver activity on the nitrogen-13 images

    D. Scaling artifact from GI activity on the rubidium-82 images

26. Which of the following cardiac PET imaging parameters has been proposed as a marker of myocardial viability?

    A. Rate of washout of ^{11}C-hydroxyephedrine from 15 minutes to 2 hours following tracer injection

    B. Retention of rubidium-82 activity on PET images obtained 3 to 7 minutes following IV tracer injection

    C. The second (slower) delayed rate of clearance of carbon-11 activity (k_2) following the IV injection of carbon-11 acetate

    D. Rate of washout of oxygen-15 water from the myocardium

27. Rest and adenosine stress rubidium-82 cardiac PET perfusion images are obtained in a 58-year-old man with the metabolic syndrome. The rest perfusion images demonstrate homogeneous tracer uptake. No regional perfusion defects are noted on the stress perfusion images, and there is no ischemic dilation of the ventricle with stress. However, there is a progressive diminution of tracer uptake from the base of heart to the apex on the stress images. Regional wall motion is normal at rest and with stress; the rest left ventricular ejection fraction (LVEF) is 57% and the stress LVEF is 62%. These findings suggest:

    A. Diffuse preclinical atherosclerotic disease of the coronary arteries.

    B. Mild systemic hypertension.

    C. Severe, proximal triple-vessel atherosclerotic disease.

    D. Apical hypertrophy with focal myocardial fibrosis.

28. Regadenoson stress/rest rubidium-82 PET perfusion images (Fig. 6.5A), along with fused rubidium-82 emission and CT transmission images (Fig. 6.5B, C), from an 82-year-old man with chest pain are shown in Figure 6.5. Which of the following best describes the findings?

    A. Reversible perfusion defect, right coronary distribution

    B. Normal study, transmission–emission mismatch on stress images

    C. Normal study, transmission–emission mismatch on rest images

    D. Reversible perfusion defect, right coronary distribution with transmission–emission mismatch on the rest images

29. Which of the following statements best describes the behavior of nitrogen-13 ammonia?

    A. $^{13}NH_3$ crosses the myocyte cell membrane as $^{13}NH_4^+$, via the Na^+–K^+ ATPase-dependent transporter protein.

    B. $^{13}NH_3$ passively crosses the cell membrane and mitochondrial membrane; the tracer is then trapped within mitochondria as $^{13}NH_4^+$.

    C. $^{13}NH_3$ passively crosses the myocyte cell membrane and transiently resides within the cytosol; when vascular $^{13}NH_3$ levels decline as a result of renal excretion, there is back diffusion of the tracer into the vascular compartment.

    D. $^{13}NH_3$ passively crosses the myocyte cell membrane; once within the cytosol of the cell, it is metabolically trapped as glutamine via the glutamine synthase reaction.

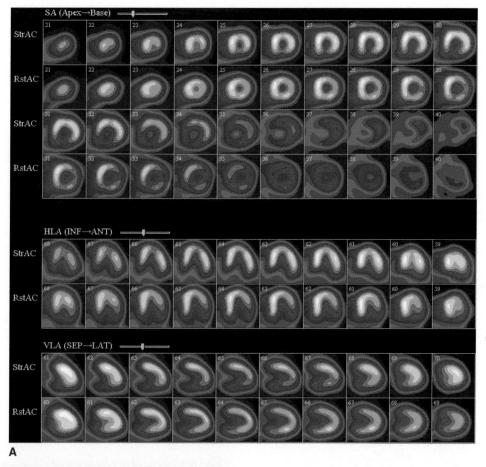

A

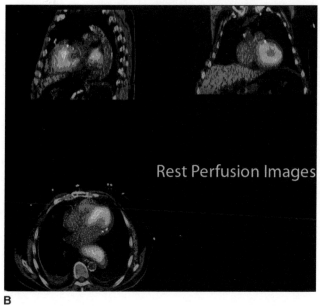

B

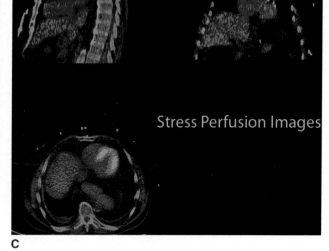

C

Figure 6.5A,B,C

30. Which of the following tracers used to assess the sympathetic nervous system of the heart with PET imaging predominantly reflects activity of the uptake-1 mechanism?

A. ^{11}C-epinephrine

B. ^{11}C-hydroxyephedrine

C. ^{13}F-6-fluorodopamine

D. ^{13}F-fluoronorepinephrine

ANSWERS

1. ANSWER: C. Rubidium-82 chloride is a short-lived (half-life = 76 seconds) radioactive analog of potassium that relies upon the Na^+–K^+ ATPase transporter for cellular uptake. Rubidium-82 is eluted from a small portable generator in which strontium-82, the "parent" radionuclide, is absorbed onto a SnO_2 column. When strontium-82 decays (half-life = 25 days), the "daughter" radionuclide rubidium-82 can be washed (eluted) off the column using normal saline. The column also contains strontium-85, a radionuclide (half-life = 65 days) that is generated as a by-product during the production of strontium-82. Problems with the generator column can release both strontium-82 and strontium-85 into the eluate. These radionuclide contaminants are tested for on a daily basis by examining the first eluted sample of the day.

2. ANSWER: B. ^{11}C-acetate is a marker of myocardial oxidative substrate metabolism. Following the uptake of ^{11}C-acetate by the myocardium, initial rates of clearance of carbon-11 activity from the tissue quantitatively reflect oxidative substrate flux through the tricarboxylic acid cycle. In clinical studies of patients with CAD, rates of ^{11}C-acetate clearance have proven useful for identifying dysfunctional myocardial segments which will exhibit an improvement in function following revascularization. Because ^{11}C-acetate has a high first-pass myocardial extraction fraction, images obtained early following tracer injection can also be used to measure regional tissue blood flow, in mL/min/g tissue. FDG is a tracer of myocardial glucose metabolism, while ^{11}C-hydroxyephedrine is used to depict sympathetic innervation of the myocardium. ^{11}C-heptagluconate is a tracer of myocardial fatty acid utilization.

3. ANSWER: D. Oxygen-15 water is a freely diffusible tracer of myocardial blood flow whose net tissue uptake is near unity even at hyperemic blood flows. For each of the other tracers, net tissue uptake gets progressively smaller for each unit increase in tissue blood flow. As a result, linearity is lost and tracer uptake no longer reflects flow. This roll off or plateau effect is a greater problem with technetium-99m tracers especially when performed in conjunction with pharmacologic stress, which has a greater increase in coronary blood flow relative to exercise.

4. ANSWER: A. The cardiac PET images depict severe matching perfusion and metabolic defects in the anteroapical and basal inferior regions, consistent with myocardial infarction. On delayed contrast-enhanced magnetic resonance images, an increase in signal intensity is typically found in areas of nonviable tissue (fibrosis or scar) and would be consistent with the infarction noted on the PET images. By contrast, postextrasystolic potentiation of regional function, thallium-201 redistribution, and an end-diastolic wall thicknesses of 8.0 to 8.5 mm would all be suggestive of significant residual tissue viability and not transmural scar.

5. ANSWER: A. Because of the long half-life of thallium-201, the effective dose from protocol A is greater than that of the other options. The estimated effective dose for the stress and redistribution thallium-201 study is 22 mSv;

for the 1-day rest–stress technetium-99m tetrofosmin SPECT imaging protocol 9.9 mSv; for the 2-day technetium-99m tetrofosmin SPECT imaging protocol 13.5 mSv; and for the rubidium-82 cardiac PET study 4.6 mSv.

REFERENCES:

Einstein AJ, Moser KW, Thompson RC, et al. Radiation dose to patients from cardiac diagnostic imaging. *Circulation.* 2007;116:1290–1305.

Senthamizhchelvan S, Bravo PE, Esaias C, et al. Human biodistribution and radiation dosimetry of 82Rb. *J Nucl Med.* 2010;51:1592–1599.

6. ANSWER: B. The likelihood that a patient with a calcium score >399 and <1,000 will demonstrate a reversible perfusion defect on pharmacologic stress PET perfusion imaging is almost 50%, based upon a study by Schenker and colleagues of 695 consecutive patients with an intermediate likelihood of CAD. In this study, the coronary calcium score provided a small, but incremental benefit for predicting ischemia on the PET scan over patient age, gender, and other conventional cardiac risk factors.

REFERENCE:

Schenker MP, Dorbala S, Hong EC, et al. Interrelation of coronary calcification, myocardial ischemia and outcomes in patients with intermediate likelihood of coronary artery disease: a combined positron emission tomography/computed tomography study. *Circulation.* 2008;117:1693–1700.

7. ANSWER: C. Schenker showed that in patients with an intermediate likelihood of CAD, the annualized event rate for patients with nonischemic PET perfusion studies and calcium scores between 400 and 999 was 5% (95% confidence intervals: 1.6% to 15.5%). Coronary calcium scores provided incremental prognostic information over that provided by the assessment of myocardial perfusion alone.

REFERENCE:

Schenker MP, Dorbala S, Hong EC, et al. Interrelation of coronary calcification, myocardial ischemia and outcomes in patients with intermediate likelihood of coronary artery disease: a combined positron emission tomography/computed tomography study. *Circulation.* 2008;117:1693–1700.

8. ANSWER: D. The PET imaging shows a small fixed perfusion defect localized to the basal anterior wall. This corresponds to the loss ("jailing") of a small first diagonal branch of the LAD at the time of the intervention; following the procedure, there was a small rise in the patient's cardiac enzyme levels.

9. ANSWER: A. PET scanners that operate in the 2D mode, also known as "septa in" PET scanners, have lead or tungsten septa interposed between the detector rings. The septa serve to reduce coincidence events between detectors in a given ring and the adjacent rings, decreasing the number of scattered events. Scanners that operate in the 3D mode, "septa out," do not have interposed septa. This permits a greater number of coincidence events between detectors in differing rings, serving to increase the sensitivity of the device as well as the number of scatter events. In general, lower doses of the radioactive tracers can be used for imaging on 3D machines than on 2D machines. Use of 3D scanners is especially attractive for imaging for pediatric patients, as it can reduce the radiation exposure. Most oncologic PET imaging studies are performed on 3D scanners, in order to maximize sensitivity for detection of abnormal tracer uptake.

REFERENCE:

ASNC Imaging Guidelines for Nuclear Cardiology Procedures. PET myocardial perfusion and metabolic imaging. 2009. Available online at: http://www.asnc.org

10. ANSWER: A. While BGO crystals have the highest stopping power, their energy and timing resolution are not as favorable as the other crystals listed. Use of the newer LSO, GSO, or LYSO crystals reduces dead times and allows higher count rates, prompting their use in 3D PET scanners.

REFERENCE:

ASNC Imaging Guidelines for Nuclear Cardiology Procedures. PET myocardial perfusion and metabolic imaging. 2009. Available online at: http://www.asnc.org

11. ANSWER: C. The cold pressor test involves immersion of a hand or foot into ice water (2°C) for 2 minutes. The stress perfusion tracer is typically injected IV at 1 minute, with imaging for an additional minute while the hand or foot remains immersed in the cold water. Cold water immersion stimulates the release of norepinephrine from cardiac sympathetic nerve terminals, which in turn results in vasodilation of the coronary circulation via the endothelium-mediated release of nitrous oxide (NO). The vasodilation induced by dipyridamole, adenosine, and regadenoson is largely independent of endothelial function.

REFERENCE:

Al-Mallah MH, Sitek A, Moore SC, et al. Assessment of myocardial perfusion and function with PET and PET/CT. *J Nucl Cardiol.* 2010;17:498–513.

12. ANSWER: A. Center of rotation is a QC procedure used to assess the performance of rotating SPECT MPI cameras. It is not used for PET scanners that have a ring detector system. The other QC procedures are used to assess the performance of PET/CT scanners.

13. ANSWER: C. Use of transmission images obtained with low-dose CT for attenuation correction of cardiac PET images allows more rapid study acquisition than transmission images obtained with a rotating line source of activity. However, objects with a very high density, such as a defibrillator coil, may not be adequately characterized by the CT transmission images. The x-ray CT transmission images overcompensate for the density of the object, resulting in hot spots on the attenuation-corrected images.

REFERENCE:

DiFilippo F, Brunken RC. Do implanted pacemaker leads and ICD leads cause metal-related artifact in cardiac PET/CT? *J Nucl Med.* 2005;46:429–435.

14. ANSWER: D. The energy of the photons imaged by a PET scanner is defined by the energy released as a consequence of the annihilation of an emitted positron by its "antiparticle," an electron. The energy liberated by this event is given by Einstein's equation: $E = mc^2$, in which m is the combined mass of the positron and electron and c is the speed of light. The masses of the positron and electron are fixed, and the speed of light is constant; therefore, the energy of the annihilation photons emitted by each of the isotopes is the same, 511 keV.

15. ANSWER: C. The urinary bladder is the critical organ for FDG. For a 10-mCi dose of FDG, the urinary bladder dose is ~59 mSv. Patients who undergo PET imaging with this tracer can minimize the radiation exposure from FDG by emptying their bladder frequently after the imaging study.

REFERENCE:

ASNC Imaging Guidelines for Nuclear Cardiology Procedures. PET myocardial perfusion and metabolic imaging. 2009. Available online at: http://www.asnc.org

16. ANSWER: D. When two 511-keV photons are generated by the annihilation of a positron and an electron, they travel in opposite directions until each photon reaches its corresponding detector. If the annihilation event occurs exactly half-way between the pair of detectors, the time that it takes for each photon to travel to its detector is the same. However, if an annihilation event occurs closer to one detector than the opposing detector, the photon traveling the shortest path will reach its detector slightly faster than the other photon. "Time-of-flight" PET scanners use the slight differences in timing of the scintillation events in paired opposite detectors to improve localization of the annihilation events.

17. ANSWER: A. As a potassium analog, rubidium-82 uptake by the kidney is significant. A recent study indicates that the absorbed dose is 5.8 microGy/MBq. The heart wall is the organ with the second largest dose.

REFERENCE:

Senthamizhchelvan S, Bravo PE, Esaias C, et al. Human biodistribution and radiation dosimetry of the PET myocardial perfusion agent rubidium-82. *J Nucl Med.* 2010;51:1592–1599.

18. ANSWER: C. Hormesis refers to a presumptive protective effect of exposure to low amounts of ionizing radiation, possibly on the basis of up-regulation of molecular cell repair mechanisms. A deterministic effect of exposure to ionizing radiation is one in which the dose is related to the severity of the effect; a deterministic effect is usually characterized by a minimal dose for the effect to be observed. A stochastic effect of exposure to ionizing radiation is one in which the probability of occurrence (as opposed to severity of effect) is determined by the dose. Stochastic effects may not have an apparent threshold dose. An example of a stochastic effect is the late development of a radiation-induced malignant neoplasm.

REFERENCE:

Tubiana M, Feinendegen LE, Yang C, et al. The linear no threshold relationship is inconsistent with radiation biologic and experimental data. *Radiology.* 2009;251:13–22.

19. ANSWER: C. Visualization of a coronary arterial plaque on FDG PET images can be impaired by high background activity due to myocardial uptake of the tracer. Use of an insulin or glucose clamp as well as oral glucose loading will serve to switch myocardial substrate utilization to glucose and thus increase the myocardial FDG background activity. A low-carbohydrate, high-fat meal will favor myocardial utilization of free fatty acids, reduce myocardial FDG uptake, and decrease background activity. All of these effects maximize FDG uptake and increase the probability of visualizing the plaque.

REFERENCE:

Rudd JHF, Narula J, Strauss HW, et al. Imaging atherosclerotic plaque inflammation by fluorodeoxyglucose with positron emission tomography. *J Am Coll Cardiol.* 2010;55:2527–2535.

20. ANSWER: B. Once FDG is transported across the cell membrane via GLUT transport proteins (GLUT1 and GLUT3 for macrophages), it is phosphorylated by the enzyme hexokinase to FDG-6-phosphate. Addition of the phosphate moiety to the molecule largely traps the FDG within the cell, as FDG-6-phosphate is a poor substrate for further glycolytic or glycogen synthetic pathways. Activated macrophages may increase their expression of hexokinase up to 10 times higher than unactivated macrophages, favoring trapping of FDG within the cell. Although macrophages can metabolize fatty acids under aerobic conditions, relative hypoxia within the arterial plaque largely precludes oxidation of fatty acids. Under hypoxic conditions, anaerobic metabolism of glucose favors trapping of FDG within the arterial plaque. Glucose-6-phosphatase catalyzes the dephosphorylation of FDG-6-phosphate to FDG. Usually, this "reverse reaction" is very slow relative to the forward reaction (formation of FDG-6-phosphate). Although not described in arterial plaques, an up-regulation of glucose-6-phosphatase would increase the rate of dephosphorylation of FDG and thereby reduce the metabolic trapping of the tracer within the cell.

REFERENCE:

Rudd JHF, Narula J, Strauss HW, et al. Imaging atherosclerotic plaque inflammation by fluorodeoxyglucose with positron emission tomography. *J Am Coll Cardiol.* 2010;55:2527–2535.

21. ANSWER: C. Accurate assessment of the degree of inflammation within a plaque requires an activity measurement that is free of influence by background activity. For atherosclerotic plaques, most of the background activity is in the arterial blood itself. Following IV administration, the clearance of vascular FDG activity is time dependent. Although there is some interpatient variability in tracer clearance from the arterial blood, prior studies indicate that PET imaging of atherosclerotic plaques should be performed starting about 2 hours following tracer injection.

REFERENCE:

Rudd JHF, Narula J, Strauss HW, et al. Imaging atherosclerotic plaque inflammation by fluorodeoxyglucose with positron emission tomography. *J Am Coll Cardiol.* 2010;55:2527–2535.

22. ANSWER: A. The images demonstrate extensive reversible perfusion defects involving the left anterior, circumflex, and right coronary distributions consistent with stress-induced ischemia and small matching fixed perfusion and metabolic defects consistent with scar in the right coronary distribution. Had only a rest perfusion and FDG metabolic study been performed, extensive ischemia would not have been identified, underestimating the potential benefit of coronary revascularization in this patient.

23. ANSWER: D. Radionuclides that decay by positron emission eject the positrons from their atomic nuclei with differing kinetic energies. Positrons with higher kinetic energies travel further, on average, than positrons with lower kinetic energies before they encounter an electron and annihilate. The positron emitted by rubidium-82 has a significantly higher kinetic energy than that emitted by fluorine-18 and thus travels farther before annihilation. This results in images that appear thicker and less distinct than the fluorine-18 images.

24. ANSWER: A. In order to obtain high-quality FDG PET images for the assessment of myocardial viability, current guidelines recommend imaging under conditions in which glucose metabolism has been stimulated. Each of the four options listed is part of protocols that will stimulate myocardial glucose utilization and that has been used for clinical imaging. However, acipimox has not been approved for clinical use in the United States by the U.S. Food and Drug Administration.

REFERENCE:

ASNC Imaging Guidelines for Nuclear Cardiology Procedures. PET myocardial perfusion and metabolic imaging. 2009. Available online at: http://www.asnc.org

25. ANSWER: B. In some normal subjects, there may be a decrease in nitrogen-13 ammonia uptake in the inferolateral region of the ventricle. The reason for this observation is not known. Quantification of absolute myocardial blood flows using dynamic nitrogen-13 ammonia PET images reveals normal rest and stress perfusion measurements, and segmental wall motion is normal. It is important to recognize this normal variant in the myocardial distribution of nitrogen-13 ammonia in order to avoid mistaking this finding for a true perfusion defect.

REFERENCES:

Beanlands RSB, Muzik O, Hutchins GD, et al. Heterogeneity of regional nitrogen-13 labeled ammonia tracer distribution in the normal human heart: comparison with rubidium-82 and copper-62-labeled PTSM. *J Nucl Cardiol.* 1994;1:225–235.

de Jong RM, Blanksma PK, Willemson ATM, et al. Posterolateral defect of the normal human heart investigated with nitrogen-13 ammonia and dynamic PET. *J Nucl Med.* 1995;36:581–585.

26. ANSWER: B. The retention of rubidium-82 activity on PET images obtained 3 to 7 minutes following tracer injection has been proposed as a marker of myocardial viability, on the premise that nonviable tissue would not be capable of transmembranous uptake and retention of the tracer. On oxygen-15 water studies, estimates of the perfusable tissue index (the relative proportion of the transmural wall perfused by the tracer) have been used to estimate the relative amount of viable tissue in the transmural myocardial region. Rates of the initial rapid phase of carbon-11 activity clearance (k_1) representing the rates of oxidative metabolism of carbon-11 acetate have also been proposed for myocardial viability assessment. The second, slower rate of clearance of carbon-11 activity following the administration of carbon-11 acetate (k_2) has not been shown to reflect myocardial viability. ^{11}C-hydroxyephedrine is a marker of myocardial sympathetic innervation.

REFERENCES:

Gould KL, Yoshida K, Hess MJ, et al. Myocardial metabolism of fluorodeoxyglucose compared to cell membrane integrity for the potassium analogue rubidium-82 for assessing infarct size in man by PET. *J Nucl Med*. 1991;32:1–9.

VomDahl J, Muzik O, Wolfe ER Jr, et al. Myocardial rubidium-82 tissue kinetics assessed by dynamic positron emission tomography as a marker of cell membrane integrity and viability. *Circulation*. 1996;93:238–245.

27. ANSWER: A. Gould and coworkers have reported that a base-to-apical diminution in tracer uptake on pharmacologic stress PET perfusion images may be identified in patients with diffuse nonobstructive disease of the coronary arteries. This parallels the findings obtained in invasive studies using Doppler flow and pressure probes. The PET imaging findings may allow the physician interpreting the study to suggest the presence of diffuse preclinical atherosclerosis in patients at risk for the development of obstructive lesions.

REFERENCES:

Gould KL, Nakagawa Y, Nakagawa K, et al. Frequency and clinical implications of fluid dynamically significant coronary artery disease manifest as graded, longitudinal, base-to-apex myocardial perfusion abnormalities by noninvasive positron emission tomography. *Circulation*. 2000;101:1931–1939.

Hernandez-Pampaloni M, Keng FYJ, Sayre JS, et al. Abnormal longitudinal, base-to-apex myocardial perfusion gradient by quantitative blood flow measurements in patients with coronary risk factors. *Circulation*. 2001;104:527–532.

28. ANSWER: D. The stress and rest perfusion images demonstrate a reversible perfusion defect in the distribution of the right coronary artery. On the rest perfusion images, a modest reduction in tracer activity is noted in the basal anterolateral area of the left ventricle. On the rest rubidium-82 images fused with the CT for attenuation correction, a misalignment between the image sets is noted. This results in a spurious decrease in tracer activity in the basal anterolateral area on the rest study. By contrast, the stress rubidium-82 images are correctly aligned with the CT attenuation map, and there is no artifact in the anterolateral area of the ventricle.

29. ANSWER: D. In the blood, nitrogen-13 exists predominantly in the form of $^{13}NH_4+$. $^{13}NH_4+$ is in rapid dynamic equilibrium with neutral $^{13}NH_3$. $^{13}NH_3$ is lipophilic and crosses the cell membrane. Once inside the cell, $^{13}NH_3$ is metabolically trapped, predominantly as glutamine via the glutamine synthase reaction.

REFERENCE:

Machac J. Cardiac positron emission tomography imaging. *Semin Nucl Med.* 2005;35:17–36.

30. ANSWER: B. Myocardial uptake of ^{11}C-hydroxyephedrine large reflects the uptake-1 mechanism. ^{11}C-epinephrine is taken up by the uptake-1 mechanism, but it is also subject to monoamine oxidase degradation and storage within vesicles within the neuron. ^{18}F-6-fluorodopamine is taken up into the neuron via the uptake-1 mechanism and sequestered into storage vesicles where it is metabolized to ^{18}F-fluoronorepinephrine.

REFERENCE:

Bengel FM, Schwaiger M. Assessment of cardiac sympathetic neuronal function using PET imaging. *J Nucl Cardiol.* 2004;11:603–616.

Imaging Systemic Diseases

Brett W. Sperry and Wael A. Jaber

QUESTIONS

1. A 69-year-old male presents with dyspnea on exertion. His medical history is notable for paroxysmal atrial fibrillation, hypertension, and hyperlipidemia. On exam, he has jugular venous distention and mild peripheral edema. His electrocardiogram shows normal sinus rhythm with normal voltage. Echocardiogram demonstrates severely increased wall thickness of both ventricles, biatrial enlargement, a trace pericardial effusion, and a restrictive filling pattern. The clinical concern is for cardiac amyloidosis. What is the *next* best test?

   A. No further testing. The diagnosis is secure.

   B. Serum free light chains to assess for light chain amyloidosis (AL).

   C. SPECT study for transthyretin amyloidosis (ATTR).

   D. Cardiac MRI for transthyretin amyloidosis (ATTR).

2. The above patient is eventually referred for SPECT testing. Which radiotracers can be used to diagnose cardiac amyloidosis?

   A. ^{99m}Tc-sestamibi/tetrofosmin

   B. ^{18}FDG

   C. MIBG

   D. ^{99m}Tc-phosphate derivatives

3. What is the primary reason for the early poor diagnostic performance of nuclear studies for cardiac amyloidosis?

    A. ^{99m}Tc-phosphate derivatives were not available.

    B. Diagnostic testing was performed only in patients with abnormal echocardiograms.

    C. Early nuclear testing predated the era of routine typing of AL versus ATTR amyloidosis.

    D. None of the above. Nuclear studies have always had an excellent performance for the diagnosis of cardiac amyloidosis.

4. The above patient's whole-body planar imaging with ^{99m}Tc-PYP is shown. Which of the following is the most correct interpretation? (Fig. 7.1)

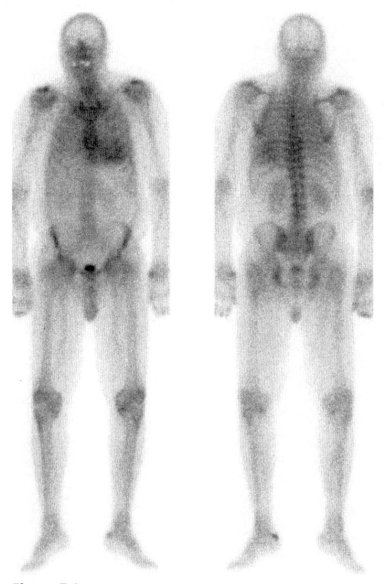

Figure 7.1

A. Moderate cardiac uptake, approximately equal to bone, consistent with ATTR amyloidosis

B. No cardiac uptake, consistent with ATTR amyloidosis

C. Metastatic prostate cancer

D. Diffuse soft tissue uptake, consistent with ATTR amyloidosis

E. Normal study

5. For this patient, a quantitative assessment is also performed by comparing counts over the heart to the contralateral chest (Fig. 7.2).

The ratio of counts over the heart compared to the contralateral chest is 1.8. What is the diagnostic utility of this ratio?

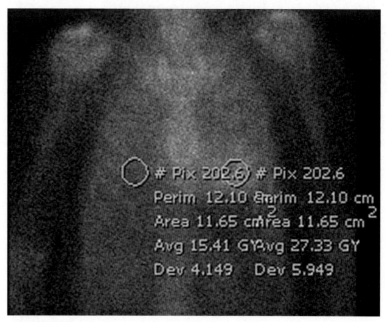

Figure 7.2

A. A ratio < 1.5 is highly sensitive and specific for distinguishing ATTR from AL cardiac amyloid.

B. A ratio > 1.5 is highly sensitive and specific for distinguishing ATTR from AL cardiac amyloid.

C. A ratio > 1 has a high negative predictive value for AL cardiac amyloid.

D. A ratio > 1 has a high positive predictive value for AL cardiac amyloid.

6. The patient's ^{99m}Tc-PYP SPECT is also shown, demonstrating the extent of cardiac amyloid infiltration. Biochemical testing for AL amyloidosis is negative. Based on these result, what is the best *next* diagnostic test? (Fig. 7.3A and B)

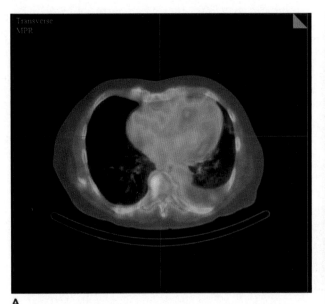 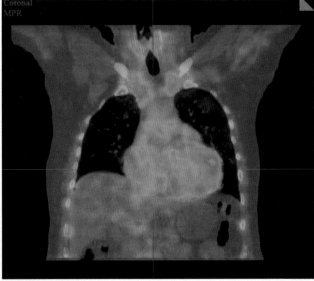

A **B**

Figure 7.3A,B

    A. Cardiac MRI.

    B. Cardiac PET.

    C. Endomyocardial biopsy.

    D. The diagnosis of ATTR cardiac amyloid is secure. Genetic testing can be considered.

7. A colleague who specializes in heart failure calls you to inquire about a ^{99m}Tc-PYP scan given a clinical concern for cardiac amyloidosis in one of her patients? She would like to know what preparation is necessary for the test. What should you tell her?

    A. No special preparation is necessary.

    B. The preparation is similar to an adenosine stress test. The patient should have no caffeine for at least 12 hours and should not eat anything for at least 3 hours prior to the test.

    C. The preparation is similar to viability imaging. The patient should fast for 6 to 12 hours, followed by a glucose load.

    D. The preparation is similar to inflammation imaging. The patient should have a prolonged fast >12 hour and have a high-fat low-carbohydrate diet before fasting.

8. A 77-year-old woman presents with dyspnea and a recent admission for heart failure. She has a history of hypertension and used to be on three antihypertensives, but her medication has been gradually tapered over the past few years due to decreased blood pressure and feeling light-headed. Currently, she is taking only metoprolol succinate at 50 mg daily and furosemide at 40 mg daily. Her exam is notable for a blood pressure of 111/72, jugular venous distention, a III/VI crescendo systolic murmur at the right upper sternal border, and a preserved A2. Her ECG is normal sinus rhythm with normal voltage. Her echocardiogram shows markedly increased wall thickness, a restrictive filling pattern, and an apical sparing pattern on global longitudinal strain (Fig. 7.4A and B). Her aortic valve leaflets are thickened with peak and mean gradients of 52 and 28 mm Hg, respectively.

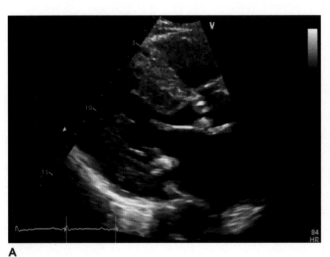

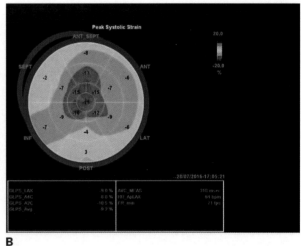

A

B

Figure 7.4A,B

What is the next best step in her management?

    A. Add back vasodilators to try to prevent further heart failure admission.

    B. Start digoxin.

    C. Refer for transcatheter aortic valve replacement.

    D. Begin evaluation for cardiac amyloidosis including serum free light chains and ^{99m}Tc-PYP imaging.

1. ANSWER: B. Amyloidosis is characterized by the deposition of misfolded proteins that aggregate into β-sheet fibrils. In the heart, amyloidosis can result from a plasma cell dyscrasia related to immunoglobulin light chains (AL) or from transthyretin (ATTR), which is further subdivided into wild-type and mutant forms. Wild-type ATTR, also referred to as senile systemic amyloidosis, typically affects white males with a median age of 70 and is often accompanied by bilateral carpal tunnel syndrome. In patients with mutant ATTR, heart failure typically develops at a similar age to wild-type ATTR. Even though the end result of cardiac amyloid deposits is a restrictive diastolic profile and heart failure, AL and ATTR are distinctly different in their initial presentation, diagnosis, and treatment. Therefore, in a patient with suspected cardiac amyloid, the investigation should begin with biochemical testing to identify a monoclonal protein in the blood or urine.

REFERENCES:

Falk RH. Diagnosis and management of the cardiac amyloidoses. *Circulation.* 2005;112:2047–2060.

Ruberg FL, Berk JL. Transthyretin (TTR) cardiac amyloidosis. Contemporary reviews in cardiovascular medicine. *Circulation.* 2012;126:1286–1300.

2. ANSWER: D. Developed initially for bone imaging, ^{99m}Tc-phosphate derivatives also accumulate in the heart after an acute myocardial infarction. The radiotracer typically accumulates several days after an infarct, possibly related to calcium overloading of the mitochondria. Subsequently, ^{99m}Tc-DPD (technetium-3,3-diphosphono-1,2-propanodicarboxylic acid) and ^{99m}Tc-PYP (technetium pyrophosphate) have both been shown to accumulate in patients with cardiac amyloidosis. More recently, ^{99m}Tc-HDP (technetium-hydroxymethylene diphosphonate) has been similarly detected in patients with ATTR. In Europe, ^{99m}Tc-DPD is the predominant agent, but is not approved by the Federal Drug Administration. ^{99m}Tc-PYP is therefore most often used in the United States, and unfortunately, there are no studies that directly compare ^{99m}Tc-phosphate derivatives.

REFERENCES:

Glaudemans AWJM, van Rheenen RWJ, van den Berg MP, et al. Bone scintigraphy with 99mtechnetium-hydroxymethylene diphosphonate allows early diagnosis of cardiac involvement in patients with transthyretin-derived systemic amyloidosis. *Amyloid.* 2013;21:35–44.

Sobol SM, Brown JM, Bunker SR, et al. Noninvasive diagnosis of cardiac amyloidosis by technetium-99m-pyrophosphate myocardial scintigraphy. *Am Heart J.* 1982;103(4 Pt 1):563–565.

3. ANSWER: C. Early studies using ^{99m}Tc-phosphate derivatives to diagnose cardiac amyloidosis were underwhelming, primarily because they were performed in an era before routine typing of AL versus ATTR amyloid. The predilection of ^{99m}Tc-DPD for ATTR was subsequently demonstrated, though the underlying mechanism remains poorly understood. Presumably, ^{99m}Tc-phosphate derivatives have a calcium-binding affinity for amyloid fibrils. Given the indolent course of ATTR compared to AL, the slower accumulation of fibrils in ATTR may be associated with increased calcium deposition.

As discussed, ^{99m}Tc-phosphate derivative have been available for decades (choice A). In addition, diagnostic testing for cardiac amyloidosis is usually performed in patients with abnormal echocardiograms (choice B), and it is unclear if the diagnostic performance would be as good in patients with normal echocardiograms who are presumably at an earlier stage of disease.

REFERENCES:

Falk RH, Lee VW, Rubinow A, et al. Sensitivity of technetium-99m-pyrophosphate scintigraphy in diagnosing cardiac amyloidosis. *Am J Cardiol.* 1983;51(5):826–830.

Kula RW, Engel WK, Line BR. Scanning for soft-tissue amyloid. *Lancet.* 1977;1(8002):92–93.

4. ANSWER: A. For an assessment of ATTR amyloidosis, whole-body planar imaging is often initially performed, followed by chest SPECT if myocardial uptake is noted. In this patient, planar imaging with ^{99m}Tc-PYP demonstrates moderate cardiac uptake, approximately equal to bone, consistent with ATTR amyloidosis. For visual scoring, cardiac and bone uptake are compared as follows:

0 = absent cardiac uptake and intense bone uptake

1= mild cardiac uptake, less than bone uptake

2 = moderated cardiac uptake, equal to bone uptake

3 = high cardiac uptake, greater than bone uptake

In general, visual scoring has a high positive and negative predictive value for ATTR in patients with suspected cardiac amyloidosis. Interestingly, the relative decrease in bone uptake on planar imaging in ATTR may not be entirely explained by competitive reduction in bone, but may also be attributed to extensive overlying soft tissue uptake, though this finding is typically better appreciated on SPECT–CT imaging.

REFERENCES:

Hutt DF, Quigley AM, Page J, et al. Utility and limitations of 3,3-diphosphono-1,2-propanodicarboxylic acid scintigraphy in systemic amyloidosis. *Eur Heart J Cardiovas Imaging.* 2014;15(11):1289–1298.

Perugini E, Guidalotti PL, Salvi F, et al. Noninvasive etiologic diagnosis of cardiac amyloidosis using 99mTc-3,3-diphosphono-1,2-propanodicarboxylic acid scintigraphy. *J Am Coll Cardiol.* 2005;46:1076–1084.

5. ANSWER: B. Compatible with the hypothesis that AL fibrils may have less calcium, about a third to one-half of AL patients will have a positive ^{99m}Tc-phosphate scan, typically with a milder degree of tracer uptake. Given this overlap, in certain situations, a quantitative evaluation of uptake may improve the diagnostic yield for ATTR versus AL. In fact, by comparing counts over the heart to the contralateral chest, a ratio of >1.5 had nearly perfect sensitivity and specificity in distinguishing ATTR from AL. More recently, this ratio has also been shown to have prognosis significance.

REFERENCES:

Bokhari S, Castano A, Pozniakoff T, et al. ^{99m}Tc-pyrophosphate scintigraphy for differentiating light-chain cardiac amyloidosis from the transthyretin-related familial and senile cardiac amyloidoses. *Circ Cardiovasc Imaging.* 2013;6:195–201.

Castano A, Haq M, Narotsky DL, et al. Multicenter study of planar technetium 99m pyrophosphate cardiac imaging: predicting survival for patients with ATTR cardiac amyloidosis. *JAMA Cardiol.* 2016;1:880–889.

Rapezzi C, Quarta CC, Guidalotti PL, et al. Usefulness and limitations of ^{99m}Tc-3,3-diphosphono-1,2-propanodicarboxylic acid scintigraphy in the aetiological diagnosis of amyloidotic cardiomyopathy. *Eur J Nucl Med Mol Imaging*. 2010;38:470–478.

6. ANSWER: D. In a study of 1,200 patients with suspected cardiac amyloidosis, ^{99m}Tc-phosphate–based imaging was combined with immunofixation electrophoresis of serum and urine as well as a serum free light chain assay. Overall, ^{99m}Tc-phosphate–based imaging had a sensitivity >99% and a specificity of 86%. When grade 2 or 3 uptake was combined with the absence of a monoclonal protein, the specificity for ATTR was 100%.

Based upon this large study, certain patients can forego an endomyocardial biopsy. Specifically, in a patient with heart failure and an echocardiogram suggestive of amyloid, the absence of detectable monoclonal protein coupled with grade 2 or 3 cardiac uptake identifies a patient with ATTR. If indicated, further genetic analysis can differentiate wild-type from mutant ATTR.

REFERENCE:

Gillmore JD, Maurer MS, Falk RH, et al. Non-biopsy diagnosis of cardiac transthyretin amyloidosis. *Circulation*. 2016;133:2404–2412.

7. ANSWER: A. In patients with suspected cardiac amyloidosis, ^{99m}Tc-PYP imaging can be performed with no special preparation. In general, planar and chest SPECT images can be obtained at 1 or 3 hours after injection. However, if persistent blood pool activity is noted on 1 hour images, delayed images at 3 hours should be obtained. In particular, SPECT imaging may be useful to avoid overlap of bone uptake, distinguish blood activity from myocardium, and better assess distribution of ^{99m}Tc-PYP uptake in individuals with positive scans.

REFERENCE:

ASNC Practice Points: *^{99m}Technetium-Pyrophosphte Imaging for Transthyretin Cardiac Amyloidosis*. https://www.asnc.org/Files/Practice%20Resources/Practice%20Points/ASNC%20Practice%20Point-99mTechnetiumPyrophosphateImaging2016.pdf

8. ANSWER: D. This patient has low-flow low-gradient aortic stenosis. However, based on the decrease in antihypertensive in the past few years, markedly increased wall thickness with normal voltage on the ECG, restrictive filling pattern, and apical sparing on global longitudinal strain, concomitant cardiac amyloidosis is possible. In fact, both ATTR and aortic stenosis predominate in elderly patients with heart failure.

Recently, when consecutive patients with aortic stenosis and at least one echocardiographic feature of amyloid were evaluated with ^{99m}Tc-DPD, 5 of 43 had increased myocardial uptake, consistent with ATTR. The coexistence of AS and ATTR may also impact prognosis. In a small study of 16 patients with aortic stenosis and ATTR, at a median follow-up of 33 months, 7 patients had died. In a study of 171 patients with ATTR, including 27 patients with low-gradient AS, short-term prognosis was poor. About a third of patients were dead at 2 years, and mortality was similar in patients with and without aortic stenosis.

Given the co-occurrence of AS and ATTR in all of these studies, ^{99m}Tc-phosphate–based imaging should be considered in patients with AS and echocardiographic features concerning for possible cardiac amyloid. An additional diagnosis of ATTR will inform prognosis and possibly affect treatment.

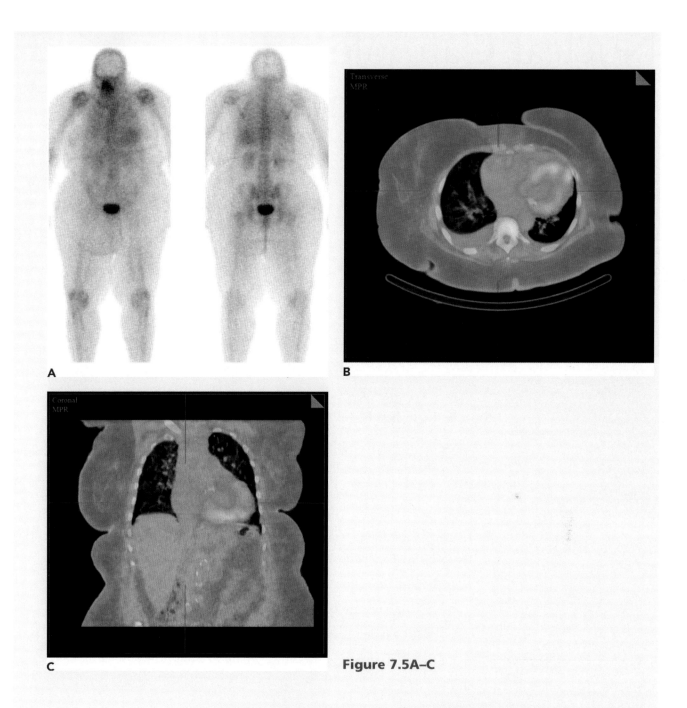

Figure 7.5A–C

For our patient, planar and SPECT imaging with ^{99m}Tc-PYP confirmed ATTR, and she was found to have the V122I mutation in TTR, a common mutation in African Americans.

REFERENCES:

Galat A, Guellich A, Bodez D, et al. Aortic stenosis and transthyretin cardiac amyloidosis: the chicken or the egg? *Eur Heart J.* 2016;37(47):3525–3531.

Longhi S, Lorenzini M, Gagliardi C, et al. Coexistence of degenerative aortic stenosis and wild-type transthyretin-related cardiac amyloidosis. *JACC Cardiovasc Imaging.* 2016;9:325–327.

Sperry BW, Jones BM, Vranian MN, et al. Recognizing transthyretin cardiac amyloidosis in patients with aortic stenosis: impact on prognosis. *JACC Cardiovasc Imaging.* 2016;9(7):904–906.

Appropriate Use in Nuclear Cardiology and Multimodality Imaging

CHAPTER 8

Wael A. Jaber

QUESTIONS

1. Which of the following abnormality on the electrocardiogram (ECG) makes the ECG uninterpretable for the purpose of exercise stress testing?

    A. Deep T-wave inversions in anterior leads

    B. Right bundle-branch block with left axis deviation

    C. Preexcitation with Wolf-Parkinson-White syndrome (WPW)

    D. Wide right bundle-branch block

2. In calculating the pretest probability for coronary artery disease (CAD) prior to ordering diagnostic testing, which of the following statements is true?

    A. Low pretest probability is defined as <10%.

    B. High pretest probability is defined as >75%.

    C. Angina type is not part of the calculation.

    D. Age > 50 results in an intermediate or high probability.

3. The global coronary artery disease (CAD) risk score is most often used to define risk in which of the following?

    A. Patient presenting with acute ST elevation myocardial infarction

    B. Patient presenting with unstable angina

    C. Asymptomatic patient—10-year risk for myocardial infarction or CAD death

    D. Asymptomatic patient—1-year risk for myocardial infarction or CAD death

4. Which of the following active cardiac conditions requires diagnostic evaluation and treatment prior to nonemergent noncardiac surgery?

    A. Stable angina

    B. History of heart failure in past 5 years

    C. Severe aortic or mitral regurgitation

    D. High-grade atrioventricular block on ECG

5. In assessing symptomatic patients with low pretest probability for CAD, the following imaging modality is considered rarely appropriate.

    A. Stress echocardiography

    B. CT calcium scoring

    C. Stress myocardial perfusion imaging

    D. CT coronary angiography

6. In symptomatic patients presenting for evaluation of possible coronary artery disease, invasive coronary angiography is deemed appropriate care in patients with:

    A. High pretest likelihood of disease.

    B. Intermediate pretest likelihood of disease and uninterpretable ECG.

    C. Intermediate pretest likelihood of disease and are unable to exercise.

    D. Intermediate pretest likelihood of disease and high calcium score.

7. In a 62-year-old asymptomatic male with low global risk for CAD, which of the following maybe appropriate care?

    A. CT calcium scoring.

    B. Stress ECG.

    C. Stress RNI or echocardiography.

    D. Testing is not appropriate.

8. A 65-year-old female, smoker with a history of hypertension presents for evaluation prior to gallbladder surgery. She denies any cardiac symptoms, and she reports that she walks few miles a day as a mail carrier. Her ECG shows normal sinus rhythm with a right bundle-branch block. Prior to proceeding with gallbladder surgery, you recommend which of the following?

    A. Exercise stress ECG since she is able to walk on treadmill

    B. Pharmacologic stress testing (myocardial perfusion imaging or echocardiography) given baseline ECG abnormalities

    C. Treadmill stress test with myocardial perfusion imaging or echocardiography since ECG is till interpretable

    D. No testing

9. A 42-year-old male presents with dyspnea on exertion, LBBB, and newly diagnosed left ventricular systolic dysfunction with an EF of 32%. What is the most appropriate way to work up this patient?

    A. No testing

    B. Exercise ECG

    C. Calcium scoring

    D. Invasive coronary angiography

10. A 73-year-old obese female with hypertension, diabetes, and a sedentary life style is being evaluated for femoral–iliac bypass surgery. Her baseline ECG was normal, and she was referred for treadmill ECG stress test. She exercised for 3.5 METs before reaching 100% of the maximal age-predicted heart rate. Your advice for this patient is:

    A. Proceed with surgery since this is a low-risk procedure.

    B. Perform CT coronary angiography.

    C. Perform pharmacologic echocardiography or myocardial perfusion imaging.

    D. Perform invasive coronary angiography.

11. A 63-year-old female patient underwent coronary artery bypass and graft surgery (CABG×4) 7 weeks ago. She presents for scheduled evaluation and reports no symptoms. She wants to join a cardiac rehabilitation program. Which of the following is appropriate care?

    A. Stress myocardial perfusion imaging to identify residual ischemia

    B. CT coronary angiography to insure graft patency

    C. Stress ECG to determine functional capacity

    D. No testing indicated

12. An 83-year-old male presents for evaluation prior to open cholecystectomy. He lives on the third floor of an apartment building and uses the stairs at least twice a day without symptoms. He has a history of hypertension and hypercholesterolemia. His baseline ECG shows normal sinus rhythm with first-degree AV block. His physical exam is unremarkable. What do you recommend prior to surgery?

    A. No testing

    B. Stress ECG

    C. Stress RNI

    D. Laparoscopic cholecystectomy

13. A 58-year-old female is scheduled for a hysterectomy for uterine bleeding and significant anemia. She had CABG 9 months earlier, had completed cardiac rehabilitation, and is symptom free. Her ECG shows normal sinus rhythm with T-wave changes. What is the best recommendation?

    A. Perform a stress ECG.

    B. Perform CT angiography.

    C. Perform stress MPI.

    D. Perform surgery.

14. A 67-year-old female presents with new onset of dyspnea on mild exertion 3 years after PCI to the LAD and LCX. She suspects her dyspnea is related to weight gain after recent bilateral knee surgery. Her ECG shows normal sinus rhythm and is unchanged from prior ECGs showing 0.5 mm ST changes in leads 2, 3, and AVF. What is the most appropriate next step?

   A. Exercise ECG

   B. Pharmacologic stress RNI

   C. Exercise stress echo

   D. Weight loss program

15. A 71-year-old male presents for follow-up 8 months post PCI of the RCA for an acute ST elevation myocardial infarction. He had >50% lesions in the first diagonal and a large second obtuse. He is asymptomatic. What is the most appropriate care for this patient?

   A. Stress RNI to assess residual myocardial ischemia

   B. CT coronary angiography

   C. Invasive coronary angiography and PCI

   D. Consideration surgical revascularization

16. A 61-year-old female with hypertension presents to the emergency department with 3 hours of chest pain that resolved after receiving 81 mg of aspirin and sublingual nitroglycerine. Her baseline ECG is normal and immediate and 6-hour cardiac biomarkers are normal. Which of the following statements regarding the use of CT angiography versus functional testing is true?

   A. Anatomic testing with CT angiography is superior to functional testing for prognosis.

   B. Anatomic testing with CT angiography leads to fewer downstream cardiac catheterizations compared to functional testing.

   C. Anatomic testing with CT angiography is associated with lower radiation exposure.

   D. Anatomic testing with CT angiography is associated with higher frequency of revascularization compared to functional testing.

17. In the PROMISE trial, which of the following modalities was NOT used for functional assessment?

    A. Stress ECG without imaging

    B. Stress echocardiography

    C. Pharmacologic stress MRI

    D. Stress myocardial perfusion imaging

18. A 68-year-old female with hypertension and diabetes presents for evaluation of dyspnea and chest pain. Her baseline ECG shows normal sinus rhythm with frequent premature ventricular complexes. Immediate and 6-hour cardiac biomarkers are normal. Based on the PROMISE trial, which of the following statements is true?

    A. Females were underrepresented.

    B. Age above 65 was an exclusion.

    C. Two-year outcomes were similar for functional versus anatomic testing.

    D. Patients with chest pain were not included in the PROMISE trial.

19. A 63-year-old male with hypertension and remote smoking has atypical angina. His internist performs a myocardial perfusion imaging treadmill stress test, which was "positive" for ischemia, and a coronary angiogram was recommended. After reviewing the patient history and performing a physical exam, you tell the patient:

    A. A cardiac coronary angiogram is appropriate since the patient is symptomatic and had an abnormal stress MPI.

    B. A cardiac coronary angiogram is appropriate if the amount of myocardium at risk is relatively large.

    C. A cardiac coronary angiogram is appropriate if his calcium score is >1,000.

    D. A cardiac coronary angiogram is appropriate if there is 1 resting wall motion abnormality on echocardiography.

20. A 59-year-old hypertensive female has dyspnea. On an exercise myocardial perfusion imaging study, she exercised to 5.1 METs and achieved 87% maximum predicted heart rate. She developed her typical dyspnea on exertion, and there were no new ECG changes. No resting or stress-induced defects were noted and her transient ischemic dilation (TID) ratio was 1.48. Her rest ejection fraction was 67%, and her poststress ejection fraction was 59%. Based on these findings, what would you recommend next?

    A. No further testing

    B. Repeat test with attenuation correction

    C. Pharmacologic stress myocardial perfusion imaging

    D. Coronary angiography

ANSWERS

1. ANSWER: C. Only WPW with preexcitation is considered an abnormality that renders the exercise ECG uninterpretable. Other abnormalities that make the ECG uninterpretable are ventricular pacing, left bundle-branch block, digoxin use, and baseline ST segment changes >0.10 mV.

REFERENCE:

Patel MR, Bailey SR, Bonow RO, et al. ACCF/SCAI/AATS/AHA/ASE/ASNC/HFSA/HRS/SCCM/ SCCT/SCMR/STS 2012 appropriate use criteria for diagnostic catheterization: a report of the American College of Cardiology Foundation Appropriate Use Criteria Task Force, Society for Cardiovascular Angiography and Interventions, American Association for Thoracic Surgery, American Heart Association, American Society of Echocardiography, American Society of Nuclear Cardiology, Heart Failure Society of America, Heart Rhythm Society, Society of Critical Care Medicine, Society of Cardiovascular Computed Tomography, Society for Cardiovascular Magnetic Resonance, and Society of Thoracic Surgeons. *J Am Coll Cardiol.* 2012;59(22):1995–2027. doi:10.1016/j.jacc.2012.03.003.

2. ANSWER: A. Based on multiple validated risk models, guidelines recommend putting patients into three pretest risk for CAD categories. These models define risk as:

High: >90% pretest probability.
Intermediate: between 10% and 90% pretest probability.
Low: between 5% and 10% pretest probability.
Very low: <5% pretest probability.

Age > 60 puts all patients, males and females, in the intermediate/high pretest probability category.

Angina characteristics are one of the elements used to calculate risk.

REFERENCES:

Diamond GA, Forrester JS. Analysis of probability as an aid in the clinical diagnosis of coronary-artery disease. *N Engl J Med.* 1979;300:1350–1358.

Morise AP, Haddad WJ, Beckner D. Development and validation of a clinical score to estimate the probability of coronary artery disease in men and women presenting with suspected coronary disease. *Am J Med.* 1997;102:350–356.

Pryor DB, Shaw L, McCants CB, et al. Value of the history and physical in identifying patients at increased risk for coronary artery disease. *Ann Intern Med.* 1993;118:81–90.

3. ANSWER: C. The global CAD risk is applied to asymptomatic individuals to identify the risk of myocardial infarction or CAD death over 10 years.

Low global CAD risk is defined by an age-specific risk level that is below average. In general, low risk will correlate with a 10-year absolute CAD risk <10%.

Intermediate risk is defined as a 10-year CAD risk from 10% to 20%.

High risk is defined as a 10-year CAD risk of >20%. CAD equivalents such as diabetes mellitus and peripheral arterial disease can also define a high-risk group.

REFERENCES:

Diamond GA. A clinically relevant classification of chest discomfort. *J Am Coll Cardiol.* 1983;1:574–575.

Expert Panel on Detection, Evaluation, and Treatment of High Blood Cholesterol in Adults. Executive summary of the Third Report of the National Cholesterol Education Program (NCEP) Expert Panel on Detection, Evaluation, and Treatment of High Blood Cholesterol in Adults (Adult Treatment Panel III). *JAMA*. 2001;285:2486–2497.

4. ANSWER: D. Active cardiac conditions are defined as unstable angina, decompensated heart failure, advanced AV block, symptomatic bradycardia, symptomatic ventricular arrhythmias, supraventricular arrhythmias (including atrial fibrillation) with uncontrolled ventricular rate (HR >100 beats/min at rest), newly recognized ventricular tachycardia, severe aortic stenosis (mean pressure gradient >40 mm Hg), aortic valve area <1 cm^2 or symptomatic, or symptomatic mitral stenosis (progressive dyspnea on exertion, exertional presyncope, or HF).

Stable angina, heart failure or regurgitating valve lesions are not considered active cardiac issues that should be addressed prior to a noncardiac surgery.

REFERENCES:

Bikkina M, Larson MG, Levy D. Prognostic implications of asymptomatic ventricular arrhythmias: the Framingham Heart Study. *Ann Intern Med*. 1992;117:990–996.

Fleisher LA, Beckman JA, Brown KA, et al. 2009 ACCF/AHA focused update on perioperative beta blockade incorporated into the ACC/AHA 2007 guidelines on perioperative cardiovascular evaluation and care for noncardiac surgery. *J Am Coll Cardiol*. 2009;54:e13–e118.

Moya A, Sutton R, Ammirati F, et al. Guidelines for the diagnosis and management of syncope (version 2009). *Eur Heart J*. 2009;30:2631–2671.

Zipes DP, Jalife J, eds. *Cardiac Electrophysiology: From Cell To Bedside*. 2nd ed. Philadelphia, PA: W. B. Saunders Company, 1995.

5. ANSWER: B. Adding an imaging modality to standard treadmill testing is considered appropriate even in symptomatic patient with low pretest likelihood of CAD. However, this is only appropriate when the ECG is uninterpretable. Calcium scoring in this population is considered rarely appropriate.

Refer to pages 16 and 17 for relevant definitions, in particular Table A and text for age, sex, symptom presentation, and risk factors relevant to each pre-test probability category

Indication Text	Exercise ECG	Stress RNI	Stress Echo	Stress CMR	Calcium Scoring	CCTA	Invasive Coronary Angiography
1. • Low pre-test probability of CAD • ECG interpretable AND able to exercise	A	R	M	R	R	R	R
2. • Low pre-test probability of CAD • ECG uninterpretable OR unable to exercise		A	A	M	R	M	R
3. • Intermediate pre-test probability of CAD • ECG interpretable AND able to exercise	A	A	A	M	R	M	R
4. • Intermediate pre-test probability of CAD • ECG uninterpretable OR unable to exercise		A	A	A	R	A	M
5. • High pre-test probability of CAD • ECG interpretable AND able to exercise	M	A	A	A	R	M	A
6. • High pre-test probability of CAD • ECG uninterpretable OR unable to exercise		A	A	A	R	M	A

REFERENCE:

Wolk MJ, Bailey SR, Doherty JU, et al. ACCF/AHA/ASE/ASNC/HFSA/HRS/SCAI/SCCT/SCMR/STS 2013 multimodality appropriate use criteria for the detection and risk assessment of stable ischemic heart disease: a report of the American College of Cardiology Foundation Appropriate Use Criteria Task Force, American Heart Association, American Society of Echocardiography, American Society of Nuclear Cardiology, Heart Failure Society of America, Heart Rhythm Society, Society for Cardiovascular Angiography and Interventions, Society of Cardiovascular Computed Tomography, Society for Cardiovascular Magnetic Resonance, and Society of Thoracic Surgeons. *J Am Coll Cardiol.* 2014;63(4):380–406. doi:10.1016/j.jacc.2013.11.009.

6. ANSWER: A. The current Multimodality Imaging Appropriate Use Criteria consider invasive coronary angiography appropriate only for symptomatic patients with high pretest likelihood of disease. Patients with intermediate risk consider a noninvasive imaging modality appropriate before proceeding with invasive coronary angiography. CT calcium scoring is deemed rarely appropriate in symptomatic patients.

Refer to pages 16 and 17 for relevant definitions, in particular Table A and text for age, sex. symptom presentation, and risk factors relevant to each pre-test probability category

Indication Text	Exercise ECG	Stress RNI	Stress Echo	Stress CMR	Calcium Scoring	CCTA	Invasive Coronary Angiography
1. • Low pre-test probability of CAD • ECG interpretable AND able to exercise	A	R	M	R	R	R	R
2. • Low pre-test probability of CAD • ECG uninterpretable OR unable to exercise		A	A	M	R	M	R
3. • Intermediate pre-test probability of CAD • ECG interpretable AND able to exercise	A	A	A	M	R	M	R
4. • Intermediate pre-test probability of CAD • ECG uninterpretable OR unable to exercise		A	A	A	R	A	M
5. • High pre-test probability of CAD • ECG interpretable AND able to exercise	M	A	A	A	R	M	A
6. • High pre-test probability of CAD • ECG uninterpretable OR unable to exercise		A	A	A	R	M	A

REFERENCE:

Wolk MJ, Bailey SR, Doherty JU, et al. ACCF/AHA/ASE/ASNC/HFSA/HRS/SCAI/SCCT/SCMR/STS 2013 multimodality appropriate use criteria for the detection and risk assessment of stable ischemic heart disease: a report of the American College of Cardiology Foundation Appropriate Use Criteria Task Force, American Heart Association, American Society of Echocardiography, American Society of Nuclear Cardiology, Heart Failure Society of America, Heart Rhythm Society, Society for Cardiovascular Angiography and Interventions, Society of Cardiovascular Computed Tomography, Society for Cardiovascular Magnetic Resonance, and Society of Thoracic Surgeons. *J Am Coll Cardiol.* 2014;63(4):380–406. doi:10.1016/j.jacc.2013.11.009.

7. ANSWER: D. Testing is not considered appropriate in asymptomatic patients with low risk. Stress ECG and calcium scoring may be appropriate care in the intermediate-risk group. In these patients, addressing the modifiable risk factors should be the target of interventions.

Asymptomatic (Without Symptoms or Ischemic Equivalent)
Refer to pages 17 and 18 for relevant definitions

Indication Text	Exercise ECG	Stress RNI	Stress Echo	Stress CMR	Calcium Scoring	CCTA	Invasive Coronary Angiography
7. • Low global CHD risk • Regardless of ECG interpretability and ability to exercise	R	R	R	R	R	R	R
8. • Intermediate global CHD risk • ECG interpretable and able to exercise	M	R	R	R	M	R	R
9. • Intermediate global CHD risk • ECG interpretable OR unable to exercise		M	M	R	M	R	R
10. • High global CAD risk • ECG interpretable and able to exercise	A	M	M	M	M	M	M
11. • High global CAD risk • ECG uninterpretable OR unable to exercise		M	M	M	M	M	M

REFERENCE:

Wolk MJ, Bailey SR, Doherty JU, et al. ACCF/AHA/ASE/ASNC/HFSA/HRS/SCAI/SCCT/SCMR/STS 2013 multimodality appropriate use criteria for the detection and risk assessment of stable ischemic heart disease: a report of the American College of Cardiology Foundation Appropriate Use Criteria Task Force, American Heart Association, American Society of Echocardiography, American Society of Nuclear Cardiology, Heart Failure Society of America, Heart Rhythm Society, Society for Cardiovascular Angiography and Interventions, Society of Cardiovascular Computed Tomography, Society for Cardiovascular Magnetic Resonance, and Society of Thoracic Surgeons. *J Am Coll Cardiol.* 2014;63(4):380–406. doi:10.1016/j.jacc.2013.11.009.

8. ANSWER: D. Diagnostic testing is not indicated in this patient since she has no active unstable cardiac condition such as unstable angina decompensated heart failure, electric instability, or severe stenotic valve lesions. Furthermore, she has no high-risk clinical features such as history of CAD, prior heart failure, cerebrovascular disease, diabetes, or peripheral vascular disease.

9. ANSWER: A. In patients with newly diagnosed left ventricular systolic dysfunction, the current appropriate use criteria consider noninvasive imaging, CT coronary angiography, or invasive coronary angiography appropriate care. Given the documented left ventricular dysfunction, determination of the cause is essential. With an LBBB, the exercise ECG is rarely appropriate care, and a calcium score alone does not provide useful diagnostic or management information.

Refer to pages 18 and 19 for relevant definitions

Indication Text	Exercise ECG	Stress RNI	Stress Echo	Stress CMR	Calcium Scoring	CCTA	Invasive Coronary Angiography
Newly Diagnosed Heart Failure (Resting LV Function Previously Assessed but No Prior CAD Evaluation)							
12. • Newly diagnosed systolic heart failure	M	A	A	A	R	A	A
13. • Newly diagnosed diastolic heart failure	M	A	A	A	R	M	M

(Continued)

Evaluation of Arrhythmias Without Ischemic Equivalent (No Prior Cardiac Evaluation)							
14. • Sustained VT	A	A	A	A	R	M	A
15. • Ventricular Fibrillation	M	A	A	A	R	M	A
16. • Exercise induced VT or nonsustained VT	A	A	A	A	R	M	A
17. • Frequent PVCs	A	A	A	M	R	M	M
18. • Infrequent PVCs	M	M	M	R	R	R	R
19. • New-onset atrial fibrillation	M	M	M	R	R	R	R
20. • Prior to initiation of anti-arrhythmia therapy in high global CAD risk patients	A	A	A	A	R	M	R
Syncope Without Ischemic Equivalent							
21. • Low global CAD Risk	M	M	M	R	R	R	R
22. • Intermediate or High Global CAD Risk	A	A	A	M	R	M	R

REFERENCE:

Wolk MJ, Bailey SR, Doherty JU, et al. ACCF/AHA/ASE/ASNC/HFSA/HRS/SCAI/SCCT/SCMR/STS 2013 multimodality appropriate use criteria for the detection and risk assessment of stable ischemic heart disease: a report of the American College of Cardiology Foundation Appropriate Use Criteria Task Force, American Heart Association, American Society of Echocardiography, American Society of Nuclear Cardiology, Heart Failure Society of America, Heart Rhythm Society, Society for Cardiovascular Angiography and Interventions, Society of Cardiovascular Computed Tomography, Society for Cardiovascular Magnetic Resonance, and Society of Thoracic Surgeons. *J Am Coll Cardiol.* 2014;63(4):380–406. doi:10.1016/j.jacc.2013.11.009.

10. ANSWER: C. The AUC for Multimodality Imaging prior to noncardiac surgery utilizes two parameters to make decisions on need for diagnostic testing: risk of surgery and patient functional class. In high-risk procedures such as vascular surgery and liver or kidney transplant, it is considered appropriate care to proceed with a stress test combined with an imaging modality. In this patient who was unable to achieve at least 4 METs, pharmacologic stress is preferred. Angiographic definition of coronary anatomy by CT or invasive coronary angiography is rarely appropriate.

Poor or Unknown Functional Capacity (<4 METs)
Refer to pages 12 and 13 for relevant definitions

Indication Text	Exercise ECG	Stress RNI	Stress Echo	Stress CMR	Calcium Scoring	CCTA	Invasive Coronary Angiography
73. • Low-risk surgery • ≥1 clinical risk factor	R	R	R	R	R	R	R
74. • Intermediate-risk surgery • ≥1 clinical risk factor	M	M	M	M	R	R	R
75. • Vascular surgery • ≥1 clinical risk factor	M	A	A	M	R	R	R
76. • Kidney transplant	M	A	A	M	R	R	M
77. • Liver transplant	M	A	A	M	R	R	M

REFERENCE:

Wolk MJ, Bailey SR, Doherty JU, et al. ACCF/AHA/ASE/ASNC/HFSA/HRS/SCAI/SCCT/SCMR/STS 2013 multimodality appropriate use criteria for the detection and risk assessment of stable ischemic heart disease: a report of the American College of Cardiology Foundation Appropriate Use Criteria Task Force, American Heart Association, American Society of Echocardiography, American Society of Nuclear Cardiology, Heart Failure Society of America, Heart Rhythm Society, Society for Cardiovascular Angiography and Interventions, Society of Cardiovascular Computed Tomography, Society for Cardiovascular Magnetic Resonance, and Society of Thoracic Surgeons. *J Am Coll Cardiol.* 2014;63(4):380–406. doi:10.1016/j.jacc.2013.11.009.

11. ANSWER: C. The AUC for Multimodality Imaging consider only stress ECG appropriate care. In the absence of symptoms, noninvasive imaging and invasive imaging are rarely appropriate care. The stress ECG will provide useful information on heart rate goals and blood pressure control on medical management and set targets for rehabilitation.

Prior to the Initiation of Cardiac Rehabilitation (As a Stand-Alone Indication): Able to Exercise							
Indication Text	Exercise ECG	Stress RNI	Stress Echo	Stress CMR	Calcium Scoring	CCTA	Diagnostic Coronary Angiography
78. • No prior revascularization	A	R	R	R	R	R	R

REFERENCE:

Wolk MJ, Bailey SR, Doherty JU, et al. ACCF/AHA/ASE/ASNC/HFSA/HRS/SCAI/SCCT/SCMR/STS 2013 multimodality appropriate use criteria for the detection and risk assessment of stable ischemic heart disease: a report of the American College of Cardiology Foundation Appropriate Use Criteria Task Force, American Heart Association, American Society of Echocardiography, American Society of Nuclear Cardiology, Heart Failure Society of America, Heart Rhythm Society, Society for Cardiovascular Angiography and Interventions, Society of Cardiovascular Computed Tomography, Society for Cardiovascular Magnetic Resonance, and Society of Thoracic Surgeons. *J Am Coll Cardiol.* 2014;63(4):380–406. doi:10.1016/j.jacc.2013.11.009.

12. ANSWER: A. The patient has a reasonable exercise capacity, >4 METs, and no clinical high-risk markers such as diabetes, heart failure, prior CAD, or peripheral vascular disease. A stress ECG or RNI is rarely appropriate care. In the absence of risk, there is no need to perform laparoscopic surgery if that is considered optimal care by the surgeons.

Moderate-to-Good Functional Capacity (≥4 METs) OR No Clinical Risk Factors Refer to pages 12 and 13 for relevant definitions							
Indication Text	Exercise ECG	Stress RNI	Stress Echo	Stress CMR	Calcium Scoring	CCTA	Invasive Coronary Angiography
71. • Any surgery	R	R	R	R	R	R	R

REFERENCE:

Wolk MJ, Bailey SR, Doherty JU, et al. ACCF/AHA/ASE/ASNC/HFSA/HRS/SCAI/SCCT/SCMR/STS 2013 multimodality appropriate use criteria for the detection and risk assessment of stable ischemic heart disease: a report of the American College of Cardiology Foundation Appropriate Use

Criteria Task Force, American Heart Association, American Society of Echocardiography, American Society of Nuclear Cardiology, Heart Failure Society of America, Heart Rhythm Society, Society for Cardiovascular Angiography and Interventions, Society of Cardiovascular Computed Tomography, Society for Cardiovascular Magnetic Resonance, and Society of Thoracic Surgeons. *J Am Coll Cardiol.* 2014;63(4):380–406. doi:10.1016/j.jacc.2013.11.009.

13. ANSWER: D. This is a patient who is asymptomatic <1 year post revascularization. The AUC for Multimodality Imaging recommend no further testing prior to any type of surgery.

Asymptomatic AND <1 Year Post Any of the Following: Normal CT or Invasive Angiogram, Normal Stress Test for CAD, or Revascularization Refer to pages 12 and 13 for relevant definitions							
Indication Text	Exercise ECG	Stress RNI	Stress Echo	Stress CMR	Calcium Scoring	CCTA	Invasive Coronary Angiography
72. • Any surgery	R	R	R	R	R	R	R

REFERENCE:

Wolk MJ, Bailey SR, Doherty JU, et al. ACCF/AHA/ASE/ASNC/HFSA/HRS/SCAI/SCCT/SCMR/STS 2013 multimodality appropriate use criteria for the detection and risk assessment of stable ischemic heart disease: a report of the American College of Cardiology Foundation Appropriate Use Criteria Task Force, American Heart Association, American Society of Echocardiography, American Society of Nuclear Cardiology, Heart Failure Society of America, Heart Rhythm Society, Society for Cardiovascular Angiography and Interventions, Society of Cardiovascular Computed Tomography, Society for Cardiovascular Magnetic Resonance, and Society of Thoracic Surgeons. *J Am Coll Cardiol.* 2014;63(4):380–406. doi:10.1016/j.jacc.2013.11.009.

14. ANSWER: B. Symptomatic patients with angina or an anginal equivalent any time post PCI need diagnostic testing with a very sensitive test. Thus, imaging studies are appropriate care. Even if such patients are asymptomatic >2 years post PCI, stress testing with imaging may be appropriate care as PCI seldom achieves complete revascularization and progression of stenosis is likely. In this symptomatic patient, recent bilateral knee surgery limits exercise capacity, and the stress ECG, which already has a lower sensitivity, is not possible and the exercise stress echo is limited. Although a weight loss program may be helpful, it is not sufficient in the presence of worsening symptoms in a patient with known CAD.

Pharmacologic stress RNI has high sensitivity and with limited exercise capacity is the most appropriate care for this patient.

Symptomatic (Ischemic Equivalent)							
Indication Text	Exercise ECG	Stress RNI	Stress Echo	Stress CMR	Calcium Scoring	CCTA	Invasive Coronary Angiography
64. • Evaluation of ischemic equivalent	M	A	A	A	R	M	A

REFERENCE:

Wolk MJ, Bailey SR, Doherty JU, et al. ACCF/AHA/ASE/ASNC/HFSA/HRS/SCAI/SCCT/SCMR/STS 2013 multimodality appropriate use criteria for the detection and risk assessment of stable ischemic heart disease: a report of the American College of Cardiology Foundation Appropriate Use

Criteria Task Force, American Heart Association, American Society of Echocardiography, American Society of Nuclear Cardiology, Heart Failure Society of America, Heart Rhythm Society, Society for Cardiovascular Angiography and Interventions, Society of Cardiovascular Computed Tomography, Society for Cardiovascular Magnetic Resonance, and Society of Thoracic Surgeons. *J Am Coll Cardiol.* 2014;63(4):380–406. doi:10.1016/j.jacc.2013.11.009.

15. ANSWER: A. This patient had incomplete revascularization by PCI at the time of an acute presentation. A stress RNI will allow assessment of the presence and amount of ischemia in the diagonal and obtuse marginal arteries and determine the need for revascularization or continued maximal medical management. CT coronary angiography in an elderly patient may be limited by calcification and will require invasive coronary angiography for PCI. Invasive coronary angiography and PCI may not be necessary if the lesions are not flow liming at the time of angiography.

Since there were no critical lesions in the left anterior descending artery or the left main artery, there is no justification for surgical revascularization without doing another test.

Asymptomatic (Without Ischemic Equivalent)							
Indication Text	Exercise ECG	Stress RNI	Stress Echo	Stress CMR	Calcium Scoring	CCTA	Invasive Coronary Angiography
65. • Incomplete revascularization • Additional revascularization feasible	M	A	A	M	R	R	R
66. • Prior left main coronary stent	M	M	M	M	R	M	M
67. • <5 years after CABG	R	R	R	R	R	R	R
68. • ≥5 years after CABG	M	M	M	M	R	R	R
69. • <2 years after PCI	R	R	R	R	R	R	R
70. • ≥2 years after PCI	M	M	M	M	R	R	R

REFERENCE:

Wolk MJ, Bailey SR, Doherty JU, et al. ACCF/AHA/ASE/ASNC/HFSA/HRS/SCAI/SCCT/SCMR/STS 2013 multimodality appropriate use criteria for the detection and risk assessment of stable ischemic heart disease: a report of the American College of Cardiology Foundation Appropriate Use Criteria Task Force, American Heart Association, American Society of Echocardiography, American Society of Nuclear Cardiology, Heart Failure Society of America, Heart Rhythm Society, Society for Cardiovascular Angiography and Interventions, Society of Cardiovascular Computed Tomography, Society for Cardiovascular Magnetic Resonance, and Society of Thoracic Surgeons. *J Am Coll Cardiol.* 2014;63(4):380–406. doi:10.1016/j.jacc.2013.11.009.

16. ANSWER: D. The Prospective Multicenter Imaging Study for Evaluation of Chest Pain (PROMISE) trial was published in *The New England Journal of Medicine*. The goal of the PROMISE trial was to evaluate anatomical testing using CTA compared with functional testing among low- to intermediate-risk patients with chest pain suspicious for CAD. The primary hypothesis of the study was that the clinical outcomes in patients assigned to anatomical testing with the use of CTA would be superior to those in patients assigned to functional testing.

The primary outcome, all-cause mortality, myocardial infarction, hospitalization for unstable angina, or major complication from a cardiovascular procedure occurred in 3.3% of the anatomical testing group versus 3.0% of the functional testing group ($p = 0.75$). Among low- to intermediate-risk patients with chest pain, anatomical testing with coronary CTA was not superior to functional testing. CTA was associated with an increased frequency of cardiac catheterization; however, it was associated with a lower frequency of invasive catheterization showing nonobstructive CAD. Anatomical testing was also associated with increased radiation exposure, downstream revascularization, and a nonsignificant increase in total costs. In conclusion, in symptomatic patients with suspected CAD who required noninvasive testing, an initial strategy of CTA was not associated with better clinical outcomes than functional testing over a median follow-up of 2 years.

REFERENCE:

Douglas PS, Hoffmann U, Patel MR, et al.; on behalf of the PROMISE Investigators. Outcomes of anatomical versus functional testing for coronary artery disease. *N Engl J Med.* 2015;372(14): 1291–1300. doi:10.1056/NEJMoa141551.

17. ANSWER: C. Patients randomized to an anatomical strategy underwent a 64-slice CTA, while patients randomized to a functional strategy underwent exercise ECG (10%) and exercise or pharmacological stress imaging (68% nuclear stress testing and 22% stress echo). Pharmacologic stress MRI was not used.

18. ANSWER: C. In the PROMISE trial, the mean age of the patients was 60.8 ± 8.3 years; 5,270 of the 10,003 patients (52.7%) were women. Furthermore, 22.6% belonged to a racial or ethnic minority group.

During follow-up, 164 patients (3.3%) in the CTA group and 151 (3.0%) in the functional testing group had a primary endpoint event (hazard ratio, 1.04; 95% confidence interval [CI], 0.83 to 1.29; $P = 0.75$).

The study participants were symptomatic outpatients without diagnosed CAD whose physicians believed that nonurgent, noninvasive cardiovascular testing was necessary for the evaluation of suspected CAD. Chest pain was the presenting symptom in >70% of patients. In fact, over 90% of patient had either chest pain or dyspnea on exertion.

REFERENCE:

Douglas PS, Hoffmann U, Patel MR, et al.; on behalf of the PROMISE Investigators. Outcomes of anatomical versus functional testing for coronary artery disease. *N Engl J Med.* 2015;372(14): 1291–1300. doi:10.1056/NEJMoa141551.

19. ANSWER: B. The 2012 appropriate use criteria for diagnostic catheterization set specific findings on noninvasive imaging in symptomatic and asymptomatic patients to justify downstream angiography and reduce inappropriate testing.

In patients who are symptomatic, ischemia on noninvasive testing involving >5% of myocardium justifies coronary angiography (indications 16 and 17). In addition, having simply an abnormal noninvasive test is not sufficient to proceed with angiography unless high-risk markers are identified.

A high calcium score also is not a justification to proceed with cardiac coronary angiography. A stress-induced wall motion abnormality in two segments or more on echocardiography is deemed sufficient to justify coronary angiography.

Suspected CAD: Prior Noninvasive Testing (No Prior PCI, CABG, or Angiogram Showing ≥50% Angiographic Stenosis)

Indication	Appropriate Use Score (1–9)	
ECG Stress Testing	**Pretest Symptom Status**	
	Asymptomatic	Symptomatic
11. • Low-risk findings (e.g., Duke treadmill score ≥5)	I (1)	U (4)
12. • Intermediate-risk findings (e.g., Duke treadmill score 4 to −10)	U (4)	U (6)
13. • High-risk findings (e.g., Duke treadmill score ≤−11)	A (7)	A (8)
14. • Other high-risk findings (ST-segment elevation, hypotension with exercise, ventricular tachycardia, prolonged ST-segment depression)	A (7)	A (9)
Stress Test With Imaging (SPECT MPI, Stress Echocardiography, Stress PET, Stress CMR)	**Pretest Symptom Status**	
	Asymptomatic	Symptomatic
15. • Low-risk findings (e.g., <5% ischemic myocardium on stress SPECT MPI or stress PET, no stress-induced wall motion abnormalities on stress echo or stress CMR)	I (2)	U (4)
16. • Intermediate-risk findings (e.g., 5% to 10% ischemic myocardium on stress SPECT MPI or stress PET, stress-induced wall motion abnormality in a single segment on stress echo or stress CMR)	U (4)	A (7)
17. • High-risk findings (e.g., >10% ischemic myocardium on stress SPECT MPI or stress PET, stress-induced wall motion abnormality in 2 or more segments on stress echo or stress CMR)	A (7)	A (9)
18. • Other high-risk findings (e.g., TID, significant stress-induced LV dysfunction)	A (7)	A (8)
19. • Discordant findings (e.g., low-risk prior imaging with ongoing symptoms consistent with ischemic equivalent)	Not rated	A (7)
20. • Discordant findings (e.g., low-risk stress imaging with high-risk stress ECG response or stress-induced typical angina)	U (5)	A (7)
21. • Equivocal/uninterpretable findings (e.g., perfusion defect vs. attenuation artifact, uninterpretable stress imaging)	U (5)	A (7)
22. • Fixed perfusion defect on SPECT MPI or a persistent wall motion abnormality on stress echo consistent with infarction without significant ischemia (<5% ischemic myocardium)	U (4)	U (6)
23. • Baseline resting LV dysfunction (i.e., LVEF ≤ 40%) AND • Evidence (e.g., PET, CMR, delayed thallium uptake, dobutamine echo) of myocardial viability in dysfunctional segment	A (7)	A (8)
Echocardiography (TTE)	**Pretest Symptom Status**	
	Asymptomatic	Symptomatic
24. • Newly recognized LV systolic dysfunction (i.e., LVEF ≤ 40%) with an unknown etiology	U (6)	A (8)
25. • Newly recognized LV systolic dysfunction (i.e., LVEF 41% to 49%) with an unknown etiology	U (5)	A (8)
26. • New regional wall motion abnormality with an unknown etiology and normal LV systolic function	U (5)	A (7)
27. • Suspected significant ischemic complication related to CAD (e.g., ischemic mitral regurgitation or VSD)		A (9)

(Continued)

Coronary Calcium Score	Pretest Symptom Status	
	Asymptomatic	Symptomatic
28. • Agatston score <100	I (1)	Not rated
29. • Agatston score 100–400	I (2)	Not rated
30. • Agatston score 400–1,000	I (3)	Not rated
31. • Agatston score >1,000	I (3)	Not rated

Indication	Appropriate Use Score (1–9)	
ECG Stress Testing	Pretest Symptom Status	
	Asymptomatic	Symptomatic
11. • Low-risk findings (e.g., Duke treadmill score ≥5)	I (1)	U (4)
12. • Intermediate-risk findings (e.g., Duke treadmill score 4 to −10)	U (4)	U (6)
13. • High-risk findings (e.g., Duke treadmill score ≤−11)	A (7)	A (8)
14. • Other high-risk findings (ST-segment elevation, hypotension with exercise, ventricular tachycardia, prolonged ST-segment depression)	A (7)	A (9)
Stress Test With Imaging (SPECT MPI, Stress Echocardiography, Stress PET, Stress CMR)	Pretest Symptom Status	
	Asymptomatic	Symptomatic
15. • Low-risk findings (e.g., <5% ischemic myocardium on stress SPECT MPI or stress PET, no stress-induced wall motion abnormalities on stress echo or stress CMR)	I (2)	U (4)
16. • Intermediate-risk findings (e.g., 5% to 10% ischemic myocardium on stress SPECT MPI or stress PET, stress-induced wall motion abnormality in a single segment on stress echo or stress CMR)	U (4)	A (7)
17. • High-risk findings (e.g., >10% ischemic myocardium on stress SPECT MPI or stress PET, stress-induced wall motion abnormality in 2 or more segments on stress echo or stress CMR)	A (7)	A (9)
18. • Other high-risk findings (e.g., TID, significant stress-induced LV dysfunction)	A (7)	A (8)
19. • Discordant findings (e.g., low-risk prior imaging with ongoing symptoms consistent with ischemic equivalent)	Not rated	A (7)
20. • Discordant findings (e.g., low-risk stress imaging with high-risk stress ECG response or stress-induced typical angina)	U (5)	A (7)
21. • Equivocal/uninterpretable findings (e.g., perfusion defect vs. attenuation artifact, uninterpretable stress imaging)	U (5)	A (7)
22. • Fixed perfusion defect on SPECT MPI or a persistent wall motion abnormality on stress echo consistent with infarction without significant ischemia (<5% ischemic myocardium)	U (4)	U (6)
23. • Baseline resting LV dysfunction (i.e., LVEF ≤ 40%) AND • Evidence (e.g., PET, CMR, delayed thallium uptake, dobutamine echo) of myocardial viability in dysfunctional segment	A (7)	A (8)

(Continued)

Echocardiography (TTE)	Pretest Symptom Status	
	Asymptomatic	Symptomatic
24. • Newly recognized LV systolic dysfunction (i.e., LVEF ≤ 40%) with an unknown etiology	U (6)	A (8)
25. • Newly recognized LV systolic dysfunction (i.e., LVEF 41% to 49%) with an unknown etiology	U (5)	A (8)
26. • New regional wall motion abnormality with an unknown etiology and normal LV systolic function	U (5)	A (7)
27. • Suspected significant ischemic complication related to CAD (e.g., ischemic mitral regurgitation or VSD)		A (9)
Coronary Calcium Score	Pretest Symptom Status	
	Asymptomatic	Symptomatic
28. • Agatston score <100	I (1)	Not rated
29. • Agatston score 100–400	I (2)	Not rated
30. • Agatston score 400–1,000	I (3)	Not rated
31. • Agatston score >1,000	I (3)	Not rated
Coronary CTA	Pretest Symptom Status	
	Asymptomatic	Symptomatic
32. • Lesion <50% non-left main	I (1)	U (4)
33. • Lesion ≥50% non-left main	U (4)	A (7)
34. • Lesion ≥50% left main	Not rated	A (8)
35. • Lesions ≥50% in more than 1 coronary territory	U (5)	A (7)
36. • Lesion of unclear severity, possibly obstructive (non-left main)	U (4)	A (7)
37. • Lesion of unclear severity, possibly obstructive (left main)	A (7)	A (8)
38. • Lesion <50% with extension partly calcified and non-calcified plaque	I (3)	U (5)
CMR	Pretest Symptom Status	
	Asymptomatic	Symptomatic
39. • Area of delayed gadolinium myocardial enhancement of unknown etiology	I (3)	Not rated

REFERENCE:

Patel MR, Bailey SR, Bonow RO, et al. ACCF/SCAI/AATS/AHA/ASE/ASNC/HFSA/HRS/SCCM/SCCT/SCMR/STS 2012 appropriate use criteria for diagnostic catheterization: a report of the American College of Cardiology Foundation Appropriate Use Criteria Task Force, Society for Cardiovascular Angiography and Interventions, American Association for Thoracic Surgery, American Heart Association, American Society of Echocardiography, American Society of Nuclear Cardiology, Heart Failure Society of America, Heart Rhythm Society, Society of Critical Care Medicine, Society of Cardiovascular Computed Tomography, Society for Cardiovascular Magnetic Resonance, and Society of Thoracic Surgeons. *J Am Coll Cardiol.* 2012;59(22):1995–2027. doi:10.1016/j.jacc.2012.03.003.

20. ANSWER: D. Despite the absence of perfusion defects, this is a high-risk scan based on the TID and the drop in EF with exercise. Based on these findings, there is concern that the patient has balanced CAD and further testing is indicated. Since the images showed uniform myocardial uptake, attenuation correction is unlikely to help identify balanced disease. The 2012 Appropriate Use Criteria for Diagnostic Catheterization set specific findings on noninvasive imaging in symptomatic and asymptomatic patients to justify downstream angiography and reduce inappropriate testing. The presence of TID (indication 18 in table below) deems coronary angiography appropriate in this patient.

Since the patient reached 87% of the maximum predicted heart rate at 5.1 METs and developed her typical dyspnea, the test achieved all the diagnostic endpoints. Pharmacologic stress testing in not indicated under such circumstances.

Suspected CAD: Prior Noninvasive Testing (No Prior PCI, CABG, or Angiogram Showing ≥50% Angiographic Stenosis)

Indication		Appropriate Use Score (1–9)	
ECG Stress Testing		**Pretest Symptom Status**	
		Asymptomatic	Symptomatic
11.	• Low-risk findings (e.g., Duke treadmill score ≥5)	I (1)	U (4)
12.	• Intermediate-risk findings (e.g., Duke treadmill score 4 to −10)	U (4)	U (6)
13.	• High-risk findings (e.g., Duke treadmill score ≤−11)	A (7)	A (8)
14.	• Other high-risk findings (ST-segment elevation, hypotension with exercise, ventricular tachycardia, prolonged ST-segment depression)	A (7)	A (9)
Stress Test With Imaging (SPECT MPI, Stress Echocardiography, Stress PET, Stress CMR)		**Pretest Symptom Status**	
		Asymptomatic	Symptomatic
15.	• Low-risk findings (e.g., <5% ischemic myocardium on stress SPECT MPI or stress PET, no stress-induced wall motion abnormalities on stress echo or stress CMR)	I (2)	U (4)
16.	• Intermediate-risk findings (e.g., 5% to 10% ischemic myocardium on stress SPECT MPI or stress PET, stress-induced wall motion abnormality in a single segment on stress echo or stress CMR)	U (4)	A (7)
17.	• High-risk findings (e.g., >10% ischemic myocardium on stress SPECT MPI or stress PET, stress-induced wall motion abnormality in 2 or more segments on stress echo or stress CMR)	A (7)	A (9)
18.	• Other high-risk findings (e.g., TID, significant stress-induced LV dysfunction)	A (7)	A (8)
19.	• Discordant findings (e.g., low-risk prior imaging with ongoing symptoms consistent with ischemic equivalent)	Not rated	A (7)
20.	• Discordant findings (e.g., low-risk stress imaging with high-risk stress ECG response or stress-induced typical angina)	U (5)	A (7)
21.	• Equivocal/uninterpretable findings (e.g., perfusion defect vs. attenuation artifact, uninterpretable stress imaging)	U (5)	A (7)
22.	• Fixed perfusion defect on SPECT MPI or a persistent wall motion abnormality on stress echo consistent with infarction without significant ischemia (<5% ischemic myocardium)	U (4)	U (6)
23.	• Baseline resting LV dysfunction (i.e., LVEF ≤40%) AND • Evidence (e.g., PET, CMR, delayed thallium uptake, dobutamine echo) of myocardial viability in dysfunctional segment	A (7)	A (8)

(Continued)

Echocardiography (TTE)	Pretest Symptom Status	
	Asymptomatic	Symptomatic
24. • Newly recognized LV systolic dysfunction (i.e., LVEF ≤40%) with an unknown etiology	U (6)	A (8)
25. • Newly recognized LV systolic dysfunction (i.e., LVEF 41% to 49%) with an unknown etiology	U (5)	A (8)
26. • New regional wall motion abnormality with an unknown etiology and normal LV systolic function	U (5)	A (7)
27. • Suspected significant ischemic complication related to CAD (e.g., ischemic mitral regurgitation or VSD)		A (9)
Coronary Calcium Score	Pretest Symptom Status	
	Asymptomatic	Symptomatic
28. • Agatston score <100	I (1)	Not rated
29. • Agatston score 100–400	I (2)	Not rated
30. • Agatston score 400–1,000	I (3)	Not rated
31. • Agatston score >1,000	I (3)	Not rated

REFERENCE:

Patel MR, Bailey SR, Bonow RO, et al. ACCF/SCAI/AATS/AHA/ASE/ASNC/HFSA/HRS/SCCM/ SCCT/SCMR/STS 2012 appropriate use criteria for diagnostic catheterization: a report of the American College of Cardiology Foundation Appropriate Use Criteria Task Force, Society for Cardiovascular Angiography and Interventions, American Association for Thoracic Surgery, American Heart Association, American Society of Echocardiography, American Society of Nuclear Cardiology, Heart Failure Society of America, Heart Rhythm Society, Society of Critical Care Medicine, Society of Cardiovascular Computed Tomography, Society for Cardiovascular Magnetic Resonance, and Society of Thoracic Surgeons. *J Am Coll Cardiol.* 2012;59(22):1995–2027. doi:10.1016/j.jacc.2012.03.003.

Rapid-Fire Review

Richard C. Brunken, Manuel D. Cerqueira, and
Wael A. Jaber

QUESTIONS

1. Figure 9.1 shows regadenoson stress (top row) and rest (middle row) $^{13}NH_3$ perfusion and ^{18}FDG glucose metabolic positron emission tomography (PET) (bottom row) images from a 62-year-old man with a history of type 2 diabetes, hyperlipidemia, and prior myocardial infarction. On a recent echocardiogram, the left ventricular ejection fraction (LVEF) was 42%.

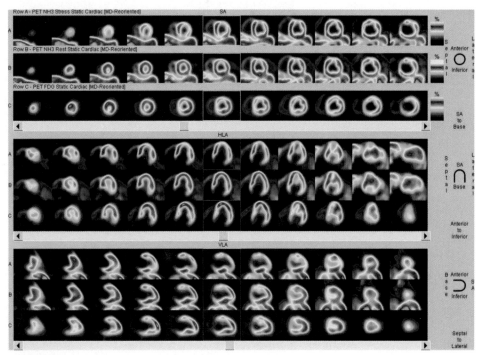

Figure 9.1

Which of the following best explains the findings on the PET imaging study?

A. Right coronary artery (RCA) infarction, with inducible ischemia predominantly in the circumflex arterial distribution

B. Inducible ischemia in the right coronary and left anterior descending (LAD) coronary distribution

C. Extensive myocardial scar in the LAD coronary distribution

D. Myocardial hibernation in the right and LAD coronary artery distributions

2. Rest $^{13}NH_3$ perfusion images (RstAC) and ^{18}F-2-fluoro-2-deoxy-2-D-glucose metabolic (FDGAC) PET images from a 59-year-old man with ischemic cardiomyopathy are shown in Figure 9.2. A recent echocardiogram demonstrates diffuse left ventricular (LV) systolic and diastolic dysfunction (LVEF = 26%), 2$^+$ mitral insufficiency, and a right ventricular systolic pressure of 42 mm Hg.

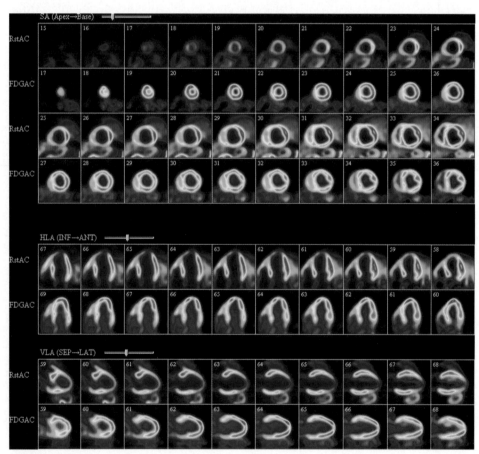

Figure 9.2

The findings on the PET imaging study are most consistent with which of the following?

A. Infarction in the distribution of the LAD coronary artery, with myocardial hibernation in the RCA distribution

B. Infarction in the right coronary and LAD coronary distributions

C. Infarction in the RCA distribution with hibernation in the LAD coronary artery distribution

D. Myocardial hibernation in the right and LAD coronary artery distributions

3. Figure 9.3 shows stress rubidium-82 PET perfusion images (StrAC) obtained following 0.4-mg regadenoson IV, along with rubidium-82 PET perfusion images (RstAc) obtained at rest. The images are from a 63-year-old man with a family history of cardiovascular disease, hypertension, and hyperlipidemia.

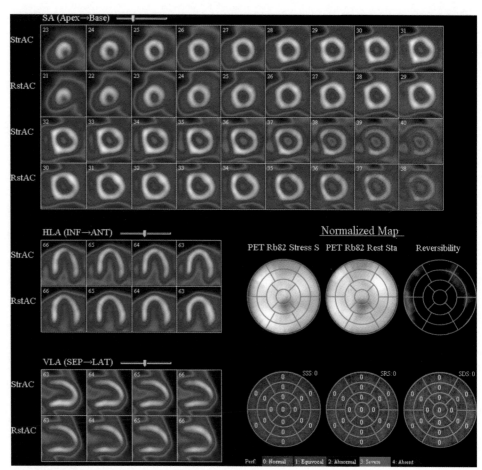

Figure 9.3

Which of the following would be the best interpretation of the PET imaging study?

A. Normal study

B. Inducible ischemia in the RCA distribution

C. Inducible ischemia in the LAD coronary artery distribution

D. Fixed perfusion defect in the RCA distribution

4. Measurements of absolute myocardial perfusion and perfusion reserve were also obtained at the time that the PET study illustrated in Figure 9.3 was performed. Segmental rest perfusion measurements ranged from 0.8 to 0.9 mL/min/g of tissue, while hyperemic measurements ranged from 3.1 to 3.3 mL/min/g of tissue. Myocardial perfusion reserve measurements ranged from 3.3 to 3.6.

What is the clinical implication of these measurements?

A. In light of the flow reserve measurements, the findings are most consistent with "balanced" ischemia (proximal three-vessel coronary artery disease [CAD]).

B. The patient has normal resting perfusion but impaired hyperemic flows due to the adverse impact of hypertension and hyperlipidemia on the coronary microvasculature. This results in lower than normal myocardial perfusion reserve measurements.

C. Normal hyperemic blood flows are present in this patient. The rest perfusion values are elevated due to the adverse impact of hypertension and hyperlipidemia on the coronary microvasculature, resulting in lower than anticipated myocardial perfusion reserve values.

D. Measured rest and hyperemic flows are normal, yielding normal myocardial perfusion reserve values. This patient's prognosis is therefore better than that of a patient with similar images but with reduced perfusion reserve measurements.

5. Regadenoson stress (StrAC) and rest (RstAC) rubidium-82 cardiac PET perfusion images obtained in a 63-year-old male for evaluation of atypical chest discomfort are shown in Figure 9.4.

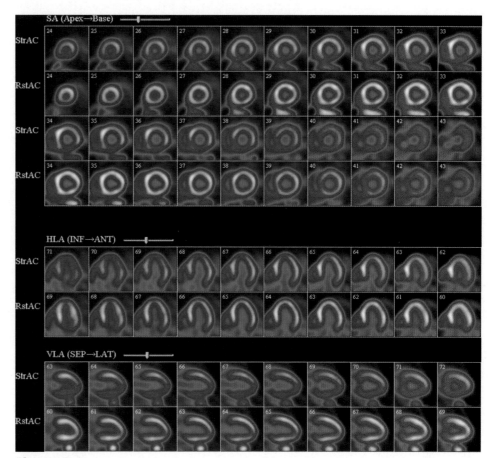

Figure 9.4

The findings on the PET images are concerning for which of the following?

    A. The images suggest "balanced" ischemia (proximal three-vessel CAD)

    B. Inducible ischemia in a median ramus distribution

    C. Inducible ischemia in a RCA distribution

    D. Artifact due to diaphragmatic attenuation on the stress perfusion images

6. Figure 9.5 shows regadenoson stress (StrAC) and rest (RstAC) $^{13}NH_3$ perfusion images and $^{18}FDGAC$ PET images from a 63-year-old woman with known CAD, LV dysfunction, prior myocardial infarction, prior percutaneous coronary intervention (PCI), hyperlipidemia, hypertension, and chest pain.

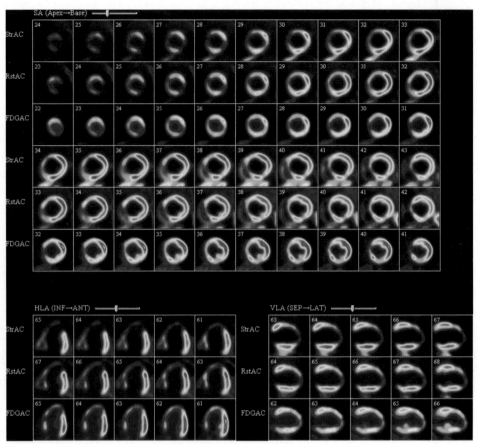

Figure 9.5

Which of the following best describes the findings on the cardiac PET imaging study?

A. Stress perfusion images demonstrate a severe perfusion defect in the LAD coronary artery distribution, with minimal reversibility on the rest images.

B. Extensive perfusion–metabolism mismatches indicative of myocardial hibernation are noted in the LAD coronary distribution.

C. A reversible perfusion defect indicative of extensive ischemia in the RCA distribution is present.

D. Both myocardial scar and hibernation are noted in the LAD coronary artery distribution.

7. A 63-year-old male with known CAD presents with chest pain and is referred for stress dual-isotope imaging. Based on Figure 9.6, a lesion in what vessel is likely to cause the abnormalities?

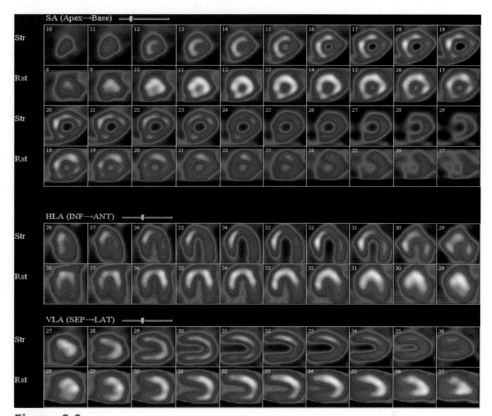

Figure 9.6

    A. Left main

    B. LAD

    C. Left circumflex

    D. RCA

8. A 79-year-old female with diabetes presents with chest pain and palpitations. She is referred for a rest/stress 1-day pharmacologic stress technetium-99m study. A resting low dose is administered and the images in Figure 9.7 are acquired. When the patient returns for the stress study, an electrocardiogram (ECG) shows a supraventricular tachycardia (SVT) with a heart rate of 150 to 175. The stress study is rescheduled 2 days later after rhythm conversion. What is the most likely explanation for the image findings?

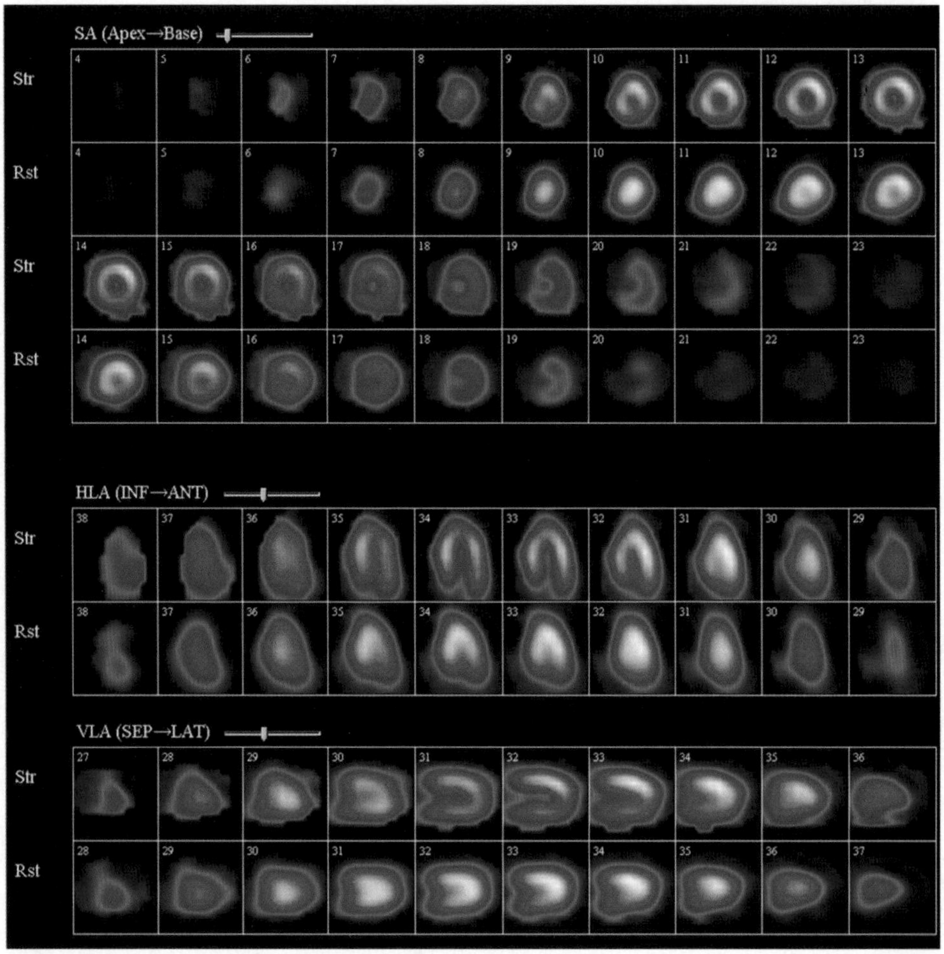

Figure 9.7

    A. Severe three-vessel CAD/TID

    B. Artifact due to the low-dose/high-dose technique

    C. Normal study

    D. Technically inadequate study

9. Which of the following cardiovascular imaging studies will give the highest radiation exposure, measured in mSv, to a patient?

    A. Diagnostic coronary angiography

    B. Computed tomography (CT) coronary angiography with prospective gating

    C. 1-day Tc/Tc myocardial perfusion imaging (MPI) study

    D. Dual-isotope thallium-201/technetium-99m

10. A patient is seen in the emergency department for chest pain and shortness of breath. He is referred for MPI. Based on the rotating projection image in the left anterior oblique (LAO) position in Figure 9.8A and the representative midcavity horizontal long-axis stress image in Figure 9.8B, what is the most likely cause of the patient's symptoms?

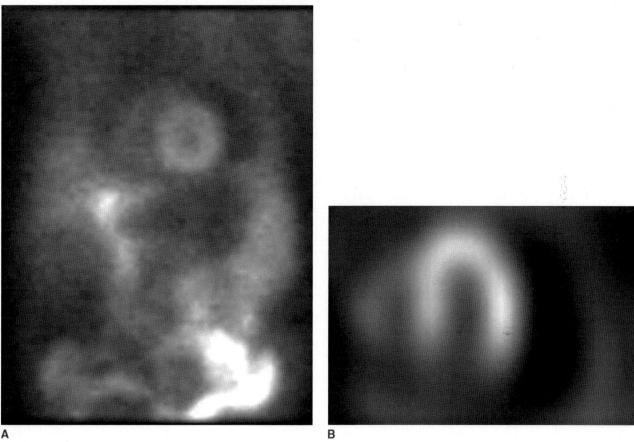

A

B

Figure 9.8A,B

    A. Pulmonary embolus

    B. Intestinal obstruction

    C. Pericardial effusion

    D. CAD

11. Which of the following radionuclide agents can be used for the detection of a recent acute coronary syndrome?

    A. Technetium-99m pyrophosphate

    B. Technetium-99m Myoscint

    C. I-123 BMIPP

    D. All of the choices

12. A patient with breast cancer is scheduled for an equilibrium radionuclide angiogram to monitor cardiotoxicity. The end-diastolic LAO view is shown in Figure 9.9. Based on the available image, what is the most likely method of red blood cell labeling that was used?

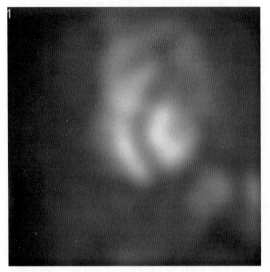

Figure 9.9

A. In vivo

B. In vivitro

C. In vitro

D. None of the choices

13. A patient with atypical chest pain undergoes an exercise stress single photon emission computed tomography myocardial perfusion imaging (SPECT MPI) study. The short-axis images are shown in Figure 9.10. Which coronary artery is most likely to have a tight stenosis?

A. RCA

B. Left circumflex artery (LCX)

C. LAD

D. Left main

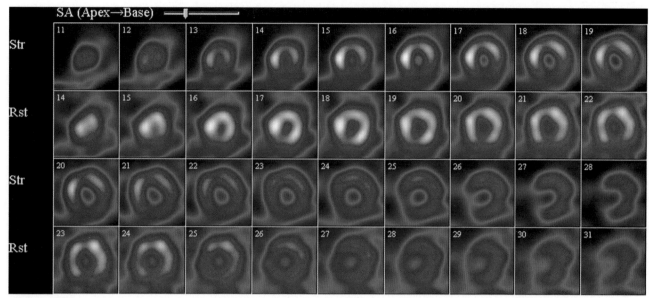

Figure 9.10

14. A female with multiple cardiac risk factors is being evaluated for atypical chest pain of 2 weeks' duration. The results of a pharmacologic stress SPECT are shown in Figure 9.11. Which combination of CAD distribution is most likely to explain these findings?

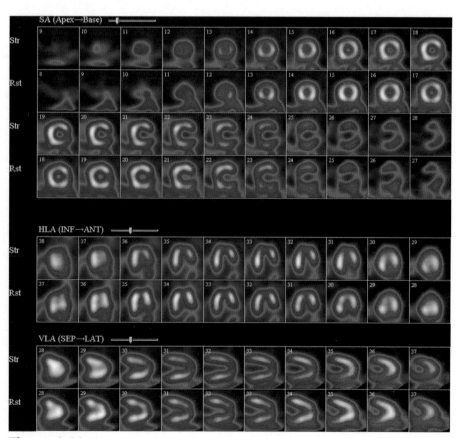

Figure 9.11

A. LAD and LCX

B. Left main

C. RCA and LCX

D. LAD and RCA

15. A 35-year-old female with atypical chest pain and no cardiovascular risk factors walks into the office for evaluation. She has a normal baseline ECG. What is the most appropriate cardiovascular test to order for this patient?

A. Stress treadmill ECG

B. Stress echocardiogram

C. CT coronary angiography

D. Stress-only SPECT MPI

16. A 56-year-old female with a remote history of CAD and bypass surgery presents with atypical chest pain and mild dyspnea on exertion. She had an uneventful pharmacologic stress dual-isotope (rest thallium, stress technetium-99m) MPI study.

Rest and stress images are shown in Figure 9.12.

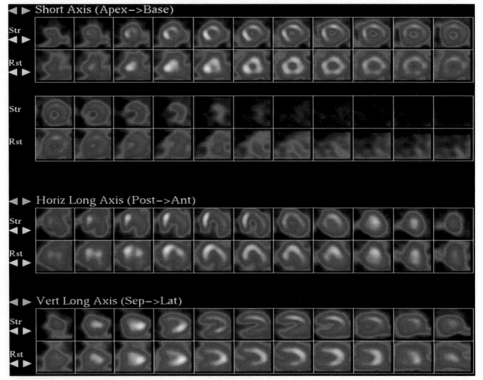

Figure 9.12

The images demonstrate:

    A. Normal with diaphragmatic attenuation.

    B. Abnormal due to a circumflex infarct.

    C. Abnormal due to a circumflex ischemia.

    D. Multivessel ischemia.

17. A 62-year-old male 10 years S/P coronary artery bypass graft (CABG) with a left internal mammary graft to the LAD artery and saphenous vein graft to the RCA is scheduled for abdominal aortic aneurysm surgery. The pharmacologic stress dual-isotope (rest thallium, stress technetium-99m) MPI study shown in Figure 9.13 demonstrates which of the following?

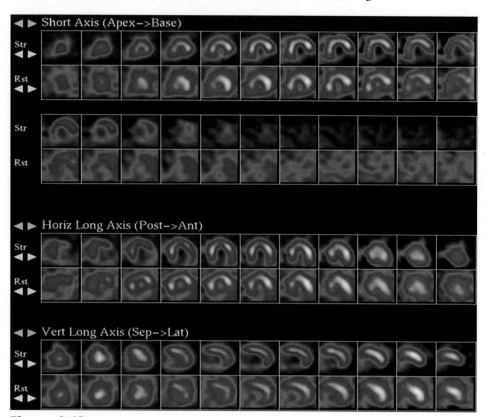

Figure 9.13

    A. Normal study with diaphragmatic attenuation

    B. RCA territory infarct

    C. Circumflex territory ischemia

    D. Right and circumflex coronary artery infarct and ischemia

18. A 53-year-old female with an old anterior wall myocardial infarction presents with heart failure symptoms and is being considered for surgical revascularization. Her LVEF is 28% by echocardiography.

A rest/pharmacologic stress rubidium-82 and FDG metabolic PET study was performed to assess the presence of hibernating myocardium. Rest and stress and FDG images are shown in Figure 9.14.

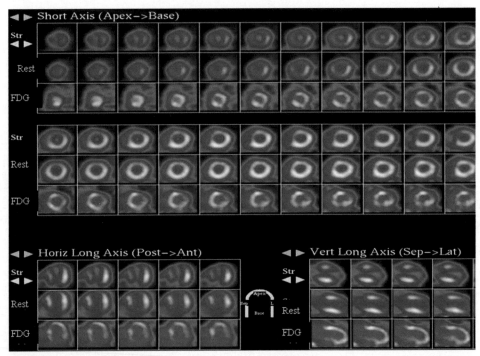

Figure 9.14

Based on the PET perfusion and metabolic study, you would recommend:

    A. Continue medical therapy and no revascularization.

    B. Medical Rx + biventricular pacing.

    C. Medical therapy and revascularization.

    D. Heart transplantation.

19. A 71-year-old male with no prior medical history presents with dyspnea on mild exertion. His baseline ECG showed normal sinus rhythm with left bundle-branch block (LBBB). He underwent a pharmacologic stress MPI with no symptoms. Rest and stress images are shown in Figure 9.15.

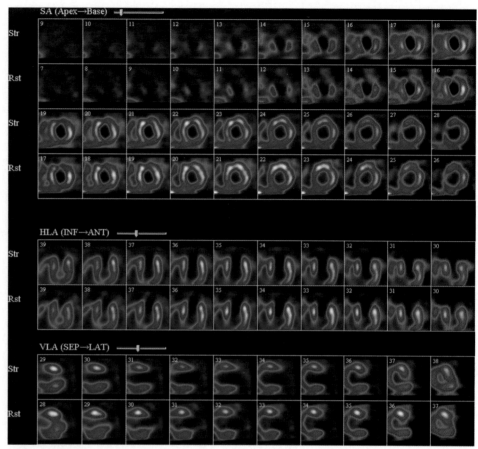

Figure 9.15

Based on these images:

   A. Breast attenuation artifact is present and a PET scan is recommended.

   B. Extensive ischemia is seen and coronary angiography followed by revascularization is recommended.

   C. No significant ischemia is seen, but hibernation cannot be excluded.

   D. An abnormal wall motion in the rest images would indicate absence of viability.

20. A 55-year-old female with diabetes, obesity, and hypertension is being considered for bariatric gastric bypass surgery. She is inactive and is asymptomatic. She underwent a treadmill stress MPI as part of her preoperative risk assessment. She walked for 5 minutes on a modified Bruce protocol and reached 78% of the predicted heart rate with significant dyspnea and 1-mm diffuse ST depression.

    Rest and stress images are shown in Figure 9.16.

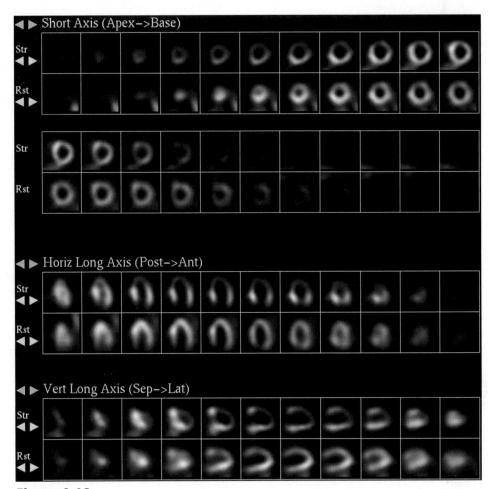

Figure 9.16

Based on these stress results:

    A. There is ischemia at a low workload and the patient is at high risk for future cardiovascular events.

    B. The test is nondiagnostic due to failure to achieve target heart rate.

    C. The MPI images show breast attenuation and therefore the test is normal.

    D. Pharmacologic stress testing is recommended to better define the extent of ischemia and risk.

21. A 53-year-old male with hypertension and atypical chest pain presents to the emergency department. He has T-wave changes on resting ECG. As part of a MPI single photon emission computed tomography study, he exercised for 10.5 METs and 110% of the MPHR. He had 1- to 2-mm ST depression in the anterolateral leads with no chest pain.

    Rest and stress images are shown in Figure 9.17.

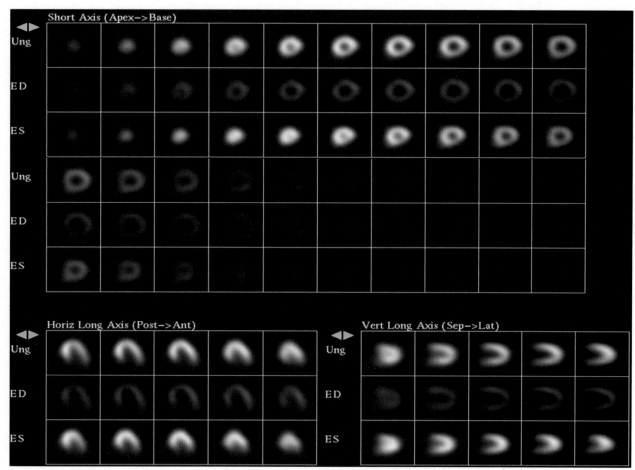

Figure 9.17

Based on the totality of the test:

A. Proceed with cath given the symptoms and ECG changes.

B. No further studies are indicated.

C. Get a CT angiography.

D. Many artifacts, order a stress echo.

22. A 56-year-old female with 2 days of chest pain several months earlier now presents with dyspnea on exertion but no chest pain. An echocardiogram demonstrated regional wall motion abnormalities with an LVEF of 40%. A baseline ECG shows normal sinus rhythm (NSR) with right bundle-branch block and small q waves in leads 2 and AVF.

A rest/pharmacologic stress rubidium-82 PET with metabolic imaging for hibernation was ordered.

FDG (*bottom row*), rest (*middle row*), and stress (*top row*) images are shown in Figure 9.18.

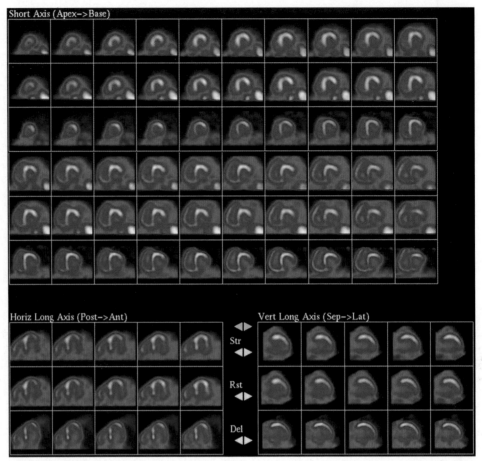

Figure 9.18

Based on the images:

    A. There is evidence of hibernation in the RCA territory and coronary angiography is warranted.

    B. There is evidence of "scar" in the inferior wall.

    C. The right ventricle is normal.

    D. Dobutamine echocardiography is needed to assess hibernating myocardium.

23. A 63-year-old male with CAD (total occlusion of the proximal LAD artery) presents for evaluation of atypical chest pain. He had a single photon emission computed tomography myocardial perfusion imaging (SPECT MPI) study done and was told that his "cardiac muscle is dead." Given the chest pain, your surgical colleague referred him for a PET study with FDG images for evaluation of hibernation.

FDG (*bottom row*), rest (*middle row*), and stress (*top row*) images are shown in Figure 9.19.

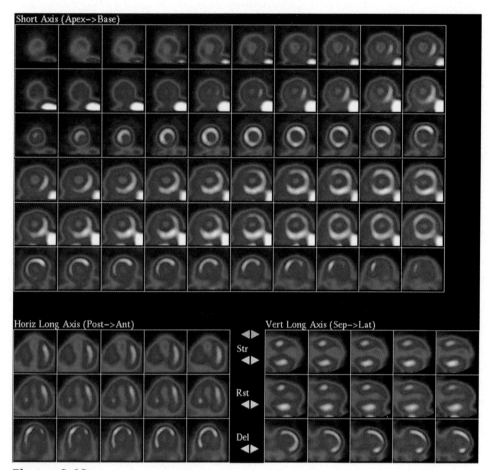

Figure 9.19

Based on the images, you recommended:

A. This patient has a reasonable chance for recovery of global LV function postrevascularization.

B. Although there is a small amount of ischemia present, revascularization is not beneficial.

C. Test needs to be repeated with delayed thallium imaging to better identify hibernation.

D. Only in patients with very severe LV dysfunction and hibernation is revascularization helpful.

24. When evaluating a patient with severe coronary disease and LV dysfunction for possible coronary artery bypass surgery and only technetium-99m tracers are available, what is the role of nitrates-enhanced technetium-99m sestamibi test to evaluate for hibernating myocardium?

    A. It has a lower positive predictive value for recovery of LV function than thallium rest/redistribution.

    B. It has a lower negative predictive value for recovery of LV function than thallium rest/redistribution scan.

    C. Sestamibi does not redistribute and should not be used for evaluation of hibernation.

    D. This is a test that could be used in this situation with a reasonable yield in terms of predicting LV recovery.

25. A patient presents for evaluation of severe LV dysfunction and CAD. He is scheduled for bypass surgery. He and his family are very concerned about "LV dysfunction" and "his pump failing." What is the best test to predict improvement of LV function and survival?

    A. There is no advantage of one test over another.

    B. Tests with high sensitivity are best suited at answering the question.

    C. Improvement in contractility on high-dose dobutamine echocardiography is very sensitive for recovery of contractile function.

    D. Revascularization improves survival and LV function, and there is no need for further testing.

26. The argument for MPI in asymptomatic diabetics is based on:

    A. Patients with diabetes are at a higher risk for development of cardiovascular disease.

    B. Cardiovascular disease is the leading cause of morbidity and mortality in diabetics.

    C. Myocardial ischemia is more likely to be silent in diabetics.

    D. Diabetic patients who sustain a myocardial infarction are at higher risk for mortality than nondiabetic patients.

    E. All of the choices.

27. Patients with diabetes have:

    A. Higher calcium score than patients without diabetes.

    B. Higher calcium score than patients without diabetes but lower mortality.

    C. Lower calcium score than nondiabetic patients, but a higher mortality.

    D. No relation between calcium score, diabetes, and mortality.

28. Patients with diabetes and zero calcium score demonstrate:

    A. Higher risk of mortality than patients without diabetes and zero calcium score.

    B. Similar risk of mortality than patients without diabetes and zero calcium score.

    C. No relationship between calcium score and mortality in this population.

    D. The need for further risk stratification with nuclear stress testing.

29. When performing adenosine or regadenoson MPI on patients with diabetes, vasodilator pharmacologic stress is expected to have:

    A. An increase in heart rate that is more pronounced than on patients without diabetes.

    B. A blunted heart rate response as compared to patients without diabetes.

    C. No relationship between blood sugar on the day of the test and heart rate response.

    D. No relationship between heart rate response and prognosis.

30. The presence of cardiac autonomic neuropathy in diabetic patients is associated with:

    A. An increase in the risk of heart failure progression.

    B. Increased incidence of diastolic dysfunction.

    C. Increased presence of silent ischemia.

    D. Impaired myocardial flow reserve.

    E. All of the choices.

31. Which of the following is the best advantage of cadmium–zinc–telluride (CZT) detectors:

    A. Improvement in energy and spatial resolution of single photon emission computed tomography (SPECT) images.

    B. Cheaper detectors.

    C. Single-view acquisition to improve sensitivity.

    D. Parallel design allowing higher count statistics.

32. The presence of calcium in a coronary artery as detected on computed tomography scans is:

    A. The reflection of an early stage in the inflammatory process.

    B. Highly sensitive but a poorly specific indicator for the presence of atherosclerosis.

    C. Correlates well with the extent of the atherosclerotic plaque burden.

    D. Often related to presence of symptoms of angina.

33. When performing multidetector CT (MDCT) coronary calcium scoring:

    A. Contrast media is needed.

    B. A slice thickness of 1 mm is needed.

    C. Radiation dose <3 mSv is recommended.

    D. It is only recommended for patients with high likelihood for CAD.

34. When coronary calcium score (CAC) is utilized in risk assessment of asymptomatic patients:

    A. A low calcium score does not add to the risk score provided by the Framingham risk score.

    B. A high calcium score does not provide incremental risk stratification to traditional risk markers.

    C. CAC is useful to reclassify patients' risk, but it has not been validated in ethnic minorities.

    D. A zero calcium score predicts very low risk irrespective of the traditional risk factors.

35. A very high CAC > 1,000:

  A. Is generally equivalent in terms of risk prediction to a very abnormal MPI SPECT scan.

  B. Predicts very poor outcomes only in symptomatic patients.

  C. Predicts hard events at a rate worse than that seen with very abnormal MPI SPECT scans.

  D. Predicts long-term events but not short-term events.

36. When using complementary information from coronary calcium scoring and MPI SPECT:

  A. Patients with normal SPECT but high CAC score have a low event rate.

  B. Patients with abnormal SPECT but low CAC have a high event rate.

  C. No complementary interaction is found between the two modalities.

  D. Calcium scoring should be done only after an abnormal SPECT MPI.

37. In asymptomatic patients undergoing PET MPI and coronary calcium scoring:

  A. A normal MPI predicts good outcomes irrespective of the CAC score.

  B. A normal MPI and a CAC > 1,000 are associated with very high event rates.

  C. A normal MPI and a CAC < 100 are associated with moderate event rates.

  D. CAC adds to PET MPI risk stratification only in patients with a CAC between 400 and 1,000.

38. When comparing radiation exposure from a typical technetium-based SPECT MPI to a typical rubidium-82– or NH_3–based PET MPI:

  A. PET-based MPI exposes patients to a higher radiation dose.

  B. PET-based MPI exposes patients to a similar radiation dose as SPECT MPI.

  C. PET-based MPI exposes patients to a lower radiation dose.

  D. Direct comparison cannot be made given pharmacologic and physical properties of the tracers.

39. Among proposed tools to reduce radiation dose during SPECT MPI is/are:

    A. Stress-only protocols.

    B. New image reconstruction software.

    C. High-efficiency SPECT cameras.

    D. Minimizing repeat tests in normal patients.

    E. All of the choices.

40. In studies assessing the sensitivity of SPECT MPI in patients using beta-blockers:

    A. The sensitivity of the test is unaffected by the use of beta-blockers.

    B. The sensitivity of the test is unaffected by the use of beta-blockers if patients achieve high exercise capacity and target heart rate.

    C. The sensitivity of the test is only affected when using vasodilators.

    D. The sensitivity of the test is reduced.

41. Which of the following medications can be continued prior to pharmacologic stress testing without reducing sensitivity:

    A. Caffeine.

    B. Theophylline.

    C. L-arginine.

    D. Statins.

42. The cardiovascular effects of adenosine include:

    A. Potent paradoxical vasoconstriction.

    B. Increase in heart rate, due to vagal stimulation at low doses.

    C. Potential for bradycardia and atrioventricular (AV) block at high doses.

    D. Direct inotropic effects.

43. The combination of low-level treadmill exercise during vasodilator stress test has added value. Such protocols can:

A. Provide incremental information about functional capacity.

B. Increase liver activity by promoting gastrointestinal (GI) flow.

C. Eliminate artifacts in patients with LBBB.

D. Lead to underestimation of the amount of ischemia.

---

44. Although uncommon, the most common adverse event with adenosine when used for pharmacologic stress testing is:

A. Bronchospasm.

B. Third-degree AV block.

C. Hypotension.

D. Second-degree AV block.

---

45. Although uncommon, the most common adverse event with dipyridamole when used for pharmacologic stress testing is:

A. Chest pain.

B. Dizziness.

C. Headaches.

D. ST changes.

---

46. When a loop of bowel is close to the heart, which of the following is most likely to cause an artifact in the inferior wall?

A. Filtered back projection

B. Iterative reconstruction

C. Resolution recovery

D. Scatter correction

---

47. Using standard acquisition and processing, which of the following is most likely to result in normalization or scaling artifacts?

A. 1-day rest/stress in an obese female patient

B. 1-day rest/stress in an obese male patient

C. 2-day rest/stress in an obese female patient

D. 2-day rest/stress in an obese male patient

48. A patient with an extreme intraventricular conduction delay on his baseline ECG and an implantable cardioverter–defibrillator (ICD) with the slow ventricular tachycardia (VT) detection set at 130 bpm is referred for MPI. Which of the following stress protocols is least likely to result in inappropriate ICD activation?

    A. Bruce protocol

    B. Dobutamine

    C. Adenosine

    D. Low-level exercise adenosine

49. A patient with which of the following devices is most likely to have artifacts when using CT attenuation correction on SPECT or PET perfusion studies?

    A. "Full metal jacket" LAD

    B. Bioprosthetic aortic valve

    C. ICD

    D. Pacemaker

50. A 40-year-old female diabetic patient with typical anginal chest pain who is unable to exercise is referred for MPI. In an effort to keep radiation exposure at as low as reasonably achievable level, which of the following will deliver the lowest radiation exposure?

    A. Stress-only rubidium 82

    B. Stress-only technetium-99m sestamibi

    C. Stress-only thallium-201

    D. 1-day rest/stress technetium-99m tetrofosmin

51. Which of the following vasodilator pharmacologic stress agents is least likely to cause high-grade AV nodal block?

    A. Adenosine

    B. Binodenoson

    C. Dipyridamole

    D. Regadenoson

52. Centering the heart in the gamma camera field of view during single photon emission computed tomography MPI acquisition provides which of the following to improve image quality?

    A. Highest counts

    B. Greatest uniformity

    C. Lowest scatter

    D. Least attenuation

53. Which of the following camera crystal materials gives the highest counts using the same injected dose of technetium-99m?

    A. CZT

    B. Sodium iodide (NaI)

    C. Bismuth germinate (BGO)

    D. Lutetium oxyorthosilicate (LSO)

54. Technetium-99m radiotracers for MPI are excreted into the duodenum where they cause scatter during acquisition if they are close to the heart. It is common practice to orally administer materials to decrease the amount of adjacent activity. Which of the following will in general give the greatest separation between the heart and the gastrointestinal tract with the least amount of attenuation?

    A. Solid food

    B. Water

    C. Soda

    D. Coffee

55. A patient referred for a 1-day technetium-99m exercise stress single photon emission computed tomography MPI study has the resting study performed. When returning for the stress portion, he is found to be in atrial fibrillation with a ventricular response of 165 bpm and stable blood pressure. He is unaware of the fast heart rate. Which of the following options is best for patient management?

    A. Inject the stress dose as he is at target heart rate.

    B. Cancel the study.

    C. Administer intravenous beta-blocker and perform exercise stress.

    D. Administer adenosine to achieve coronary vasodilation.

56. A 28-year-old female with atypical chest pain and a LBBB on her baseline ECG is referred for an exercise stress dual-isotope single photon emission computed tomography MPI. What is the best management decision for this patient?

    A. Perform the study as ordered.

    B. Refer for exercise nitrogen-13 ammonia PET study.

    C. Refer for stress echocardiography.

    D. Refer for 1-day exercise technetium-99m tetrofosmin.

57. Halfway through stress portion of an exercise single photon emission computed tomography MPI study acquisition, the patient rolls 3 inches toward his left side due to back discomfort. The patient is in a hurry to get to his next appointment and refuses to repeat the acquisition. Which of the following is the most efficient and likely to give accurate results?

    A. Interpret the study as is.

    B. Perform motion correction.

    C. Insist on repeat imaging.

    D. Refer for stress echocardiography.

58. A patient with a distant CABG and anginal chest pain who is scheduled for emergency hip surgery is referred for adenosine SPECT MPI 3 hours after a technetium-99m aerosol lung scan, which was negative for pulmonary embolus. The surgeons will not operate without exclusion of CAD. Which of the following is the best management decision?

    A. Perform the study as requested.

    B. Reschedule the patient in 24 hours.

    C. Clear the patient for surgery.

    D. Perform adenosine rubidium-82 PET study.

59. A morbidly obese female patient undergoes a 2-day adenosine technetium-99m sestamibi study. The stress images on the second day have very low counts and a planar image of the right arm injection site shows a large amount of infiltrated dose. Which of the following repeat acquisition steps is most likely to provide diagnostic information without requiring a repeat stress study?

    A. Increase imaging time

    B. Image in prone position

    C. Use an ultrahigh-resolution collimator

    D. Administer 10 mCi of sestamibi

60. When performing a fluorine-18 fluorodeoxyglucose positron emission tomography (FDG PET) study for assessing hibernation, which of the following patient preparation methods provides the most accurate results?

    A. 12-hour fast

    B. 18-hour fast

    C. 24-hour fast

    D. No restrictions

61. Which of the following gamma camera systems is optimal for obtaining the LAO views of the heart on equilibrium radionuclide angiography or multiple gated acquisition (MUGA)?

    A. Dual-headed large field of view

    B. Single-headed large field of view

    C. Dual-headed small field of view

    D. Single-headed small field of view

ANSWERS

1. ANSWER: B. The stress $^{13}NH_3$ images demonstrate perfusion defects involving the anterior wall, apex, and apical inferior segments. Full reversibility is noted on the rest $^{13}NH_3$ perfusion images in the apex, apical inferior, and mid and distal anterior walls, while partial reversibility is noted in the proximal anterior wall. Confirmation of tissue viability in the anterior wall is indicated by preserved ^{18}FDG uptake in this area.

2. ANSWER: D. The $^{13}NH_3$ images demonstrate extensive rest perfusion defects involving the mid and distal anterior wall, apex, anterior and inferior septum, and mid and basal inferior wall. Preserved tissue metabolism is present in these hypoperfused regions on the ^{18}FDG glucose images, indicating viability. Based on the findings of the cardiac PET viability study and suitable coronary anatomy, the patient was referred for multivessel CABG and had an uncomplicated postoperative course.

3. ANSWER: A. The stress and rest perfusion images demonstrate a normal pattern of tracer uptake, without findings to suggest inducible ischemia or a fixed myocardial perfusion defect.

4. ANSWER: D. In this patient, rest and hyperemic perfusion measurements are normal, as are derived perfusion reserve determinations. Resting LV myocardial blood flow parallels tissue oxygen consumption and is generally in the range of 0.7 to 1.2 mL/min/g. Clinical studies have shown a linear relationship between rest perfusion measurements and the resting double product (heart rate × systolic blood pressure) as an index of myocardial oxygen consumption. With vasodilator stress, hyperemic myocardial blood flows generally exceed 2.5 mL/min/g, such that calculated perfusion reserves (ratios of hyperemic/rest perfusion measurements) typically are >2.5. A reduced perfusion reserve determination on PET imaging may reflect either epicardial coronary disease or microvascular disease or both. Recent studies indicate that the 1-year risk of cardiac death or myocardial infarction is significantly lower if myocardial perfusion reserve is 2 or greater, regardless of whether visually assessed stress perfusion defect scores are less than or greater than 4.

REFERENCE:

Ziadi MC, deKemp RA, Williams KA, et al. Impaired myocardial perfusion reserve on rubidium-82 positron emission tomography imaging predicts adverse outcomes in patients assessed for myocardial ischemia. *J Am Coll Cardiol.* 2011;58:740–748.

5. ANSWER: C. A reversible perfusion defect consistent with stress-induced ischemia is noted in the inferior and basal inferoseptal region of the ventricle, in an RCA distribution. Ischemia involving a median ramus distribution would be expected to involve the anterolateral and apical lateral myocardial segments. No findings such as transient dilation of the left ventricle with stress are noted on the images to suggest balanced three-vessel ischemia. Because attenuation is accurately corrected for by use of transmission images in cardiac PET imaging, artifact due to diaphragmatic attenuation is unlikely.

6. ANSWER: A. The PET images demonstrate a severe stress perfusion defect in the LAD coronary artery distribution that exhibits minimal improvement on the rest images in the apical, apical septal, and apical anterior segments. No hypoperfused myocardial regions with enhanced FDG uptake are noted to suggest myocardial hibernation. No reversible perfusion defects are identified in right coronary distribution to suggest ischemia.

7. ANSWER: C. The images show a moderately severe lateral wall defect extending from the apex to the midcavity. There is also visual transient ischemic dilation of the left ventricle with a calculated ratio of 1.33, which is increased even for a dual-isotope study.

Coronary angiography found a 70% stenosis in a large first obtuse marginal branch that was treated with PCI.

8. ANSWER: C. The images show transient ischemic dilation, but this was most consistent with the patient being in an SVT at the time of imaging with a rate in the 150 to 175 range and diminished filling of the left ventricle due to marked shortening of the diastolic filling period. In essence, this was a stress study due to the very rapid heart rate. When the patient returned for the stress study following cardioversion, the rate was in the 60s at rest with a longer filling period and the cavity is bigger. With pharmacologic stress, there was no evidence of ischemia just mild diaphragmatic attenuation. The low-dose/high-dose technique does not make the cavity appear different in size between the two studies.

9. ANSWER: D. Since the dual-isotope study uses 3 to 4 mCi of thallium-201, which has a 72-hour half-life, it will give the highest radiation exposure to the patient at ~27 mSv. The other three studies will usually result in values <15 mSv and with some of the newest systems, MDCT systems and acquisition software, maybe as low as 1 to 2 mSv.

10. ANSWER: C. The patient has a lateral and right ventricular halo surrounding the heart on the projection image (Fig. 9.8A) and can be seen on the horizontal long-axis image (Fig. 9.8B) and is most consistent with a pericardial effusion. A pulmonary embolus cannot be detected on perfusion imaging, and even though there is a distended stomach bubble below the heart, this is usually a result of giving the patient fluids to get greater separation between the inferior wall and gastric and intestinal activity that may be close to the heart. The single stress perfusion image shows uniform perfusion, and this does not definitively exclude CAD but makes it less likely.

11. ANSWER: D. Technetium-99m pyrophosphate is retained in areas of healing infarction and has been used for detection of infarcts that are 3 to 7 days old. Technetium-99m Myoscint is an antibody directed to myosin that is exposed following acute damage and detects damage earlier than technetium-99m pyrophosphate.

BMIPP is a fatty acid analog that is not taken up in areas of infarction due to cell damage. Areas of surrounding ischemia at the time of the infarction also fail to use fatty acids and may overestimate the area of actual infarction.

12. ANSWER: C. The image shows excellent delineation of the ventricular blood volumes with a very low background activity. Based on the excellent image quality, the in vitro method is likely to give the best results and is the best answer.

13. ANSWER: A. The images show a classic distribution for right coronary artery ischemia with involvement of the inferior wall from the apex to the base and extending to involve the inferolateral wall at the base. There is no evidence of infarction.

14. ANSWER: A. The study shows an apical and lateral wall infarction with periinfarct ischemia in the lateral wall. A tight stenosis in the left main would not involve the apex and spare the majority of the anterior wall and septum. Although the RCA may sometimes supply the inferolateral wall, it seldom supplies blood to the anterolateral wall, and there is no inferior wall involvement. Thus, distal LAD infarct in combination with an LCX infarction and residual ischemia is the most likely explanation for these findings.

15. ANSWER: A. With such a low pretest probability of coronary artery disease, it could be argued that no testing is needed. If testing is felt necessary, the stress ECG avoids the risks of radiation and contrast reactions. A stress echocardiogram avoids radiation and contrast, but the ECG offers sufficient accuracy in this low-risk patient that it is the appropriate first test.

16. ANSWER: C. There is a moderate perfusion defect involving the entire inferior and inferolateral wall.

Her coronary angiogram showed a patent left mammary graft to the LAD artery and severe disease of the saphenous vein graft to the left circumflex coronary artery and total occlusion of the vein graft to the RCA.

A semiquantitative map showing inferior and inferolateral ischemia is shown in Figure 9.20.

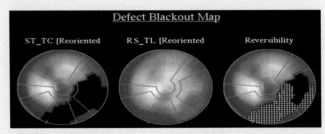

Figure 9.20

17. ANSWER: D. The patient has a severe fixed perfusion defect in the inferior and inferolateral wall with reversible component at the edges of the defect as depicted in the semiquantitative analysis in Figure 9.21.

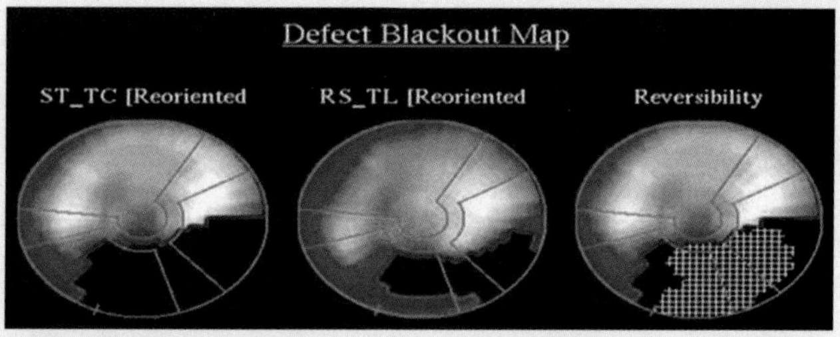

Defect Blackout Map

Figure 9.21

18. ANSWER: C. The patient has a mixture of a large area of hibernation (green arrow, Fig. 9.22) and ischemia (red arrow) in the LAD artery territory. Surgical revascularization of her LAD, first and second diagonal, was performed.

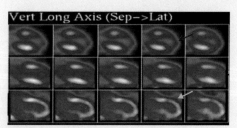

Figure 9.22

19. ANSWER: C. This scan shows a large fixed and severe perfusion defect in the LAD artery and the RCA distributions. A semiquantitative analysis of the images with polar maps is shown in Figure 9.23. The LVEF was 28%. No significant ischemia is demonstrated and coronary angiography is not yet indicated. However, if on further testing (PET or MRI) a significant amount of myocardium at risk is demonstrated (hibernation), an angiogram and revascularization would be indicated. Ischemic, stunned, infarcted, or hibernating segments of myocardium may all present as a wall motion abnormality.

20. ANSWER: A. Despite failure to achieve target MPHR, the patient had ST changes and a large area of LAD artery territory ischemia with transient ischemic dilation. The presence of defects on the stress images and not on the rest images is unlikely to be due to breast attenuation. Enough diagnostic and prognostic information were derived from this test, and therefore, there is no need for a pharmacologic stress test. Semiquantitative analysis of the images is depicted in Figure 9.24.

21. ANSWER: B. The patient had excellent functional capacity, and the MPI images do not demonstrate ischemia or infarcts. Semiquantitative analysis of the rest and stress images and comparison to a normal male database are shown in Figure 9.25.

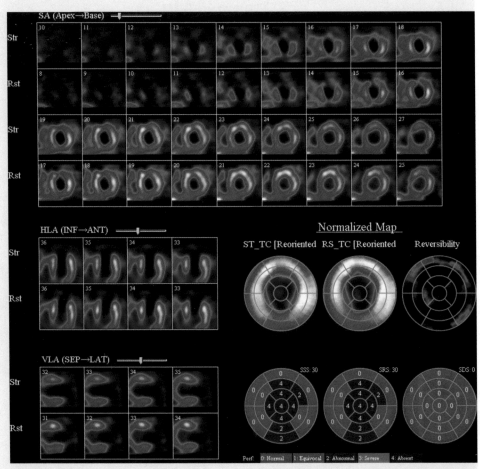

Figure 9.23

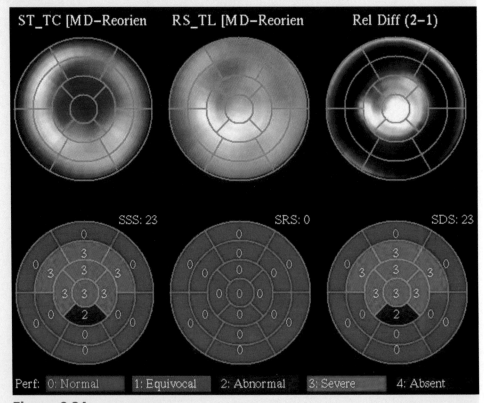

Figure 9.24

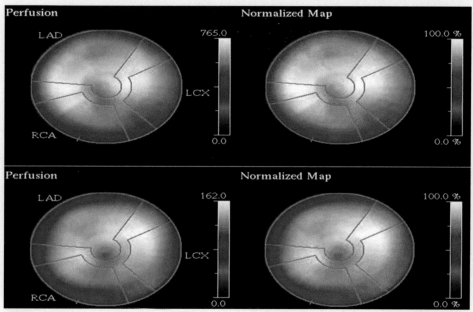

Figure 9.25

22. ANSWER: B. The rubidium images show a fixed perfusion defect with a matched defect in the FDG images consistent with scarred myocardium in the RCA distribution (see semiquantitative analysis in Fig. 9.26). In this setting, revascularization is unlikely to improve prognosis. There is intense uptake in the right ventricle consistent with hypertrophy due to pulmonary hypertension. Although dobutamine echocardiography is a more specific modality to predict recovery of wall motion and contractility, its sensitivity for hibernation is lower than PET.

23. ANSWER: A. There is a large amount of hibernation (resting defect with FDG uptake) and a small amount of ischemia (rest vs. stress). Patients with this amount of myocardium at risk are good candidates for revascularization with expected recovery of global function. PET is more sensitive for detecting hibernation than thallium-delayed imaging. Patients with very poor ejection fraction, <20%, may not benefit from revascularization even with the presence of hibernation given extensive remodeling.

24. ANSWER: D. Nitrates-enhanced technetium-99m sestamibi test is a reasonable test to evaluate for hibernating myocardium. It has a better positive and negative predictive value compared to thallium rest–redistribution (Table 9-1).

25. ANSWER: A. In a meta-analysis of 3,088 patients, no statistically significant difference in prediction of survival benefit with revascularization was detected between testing methods (see Fig. 9.27). Furthermore, improvement in survival was a function of the presence of total viable myocardium and the degree of LV dysfunction.

Improvement in contractility with a biphasic response on low-dose dobutamine echocardiography is very specific for recovery of contractile function. It is evident that a survival benefit is not seen in patients who had no viable myocardium irrespective of baseline LV function.

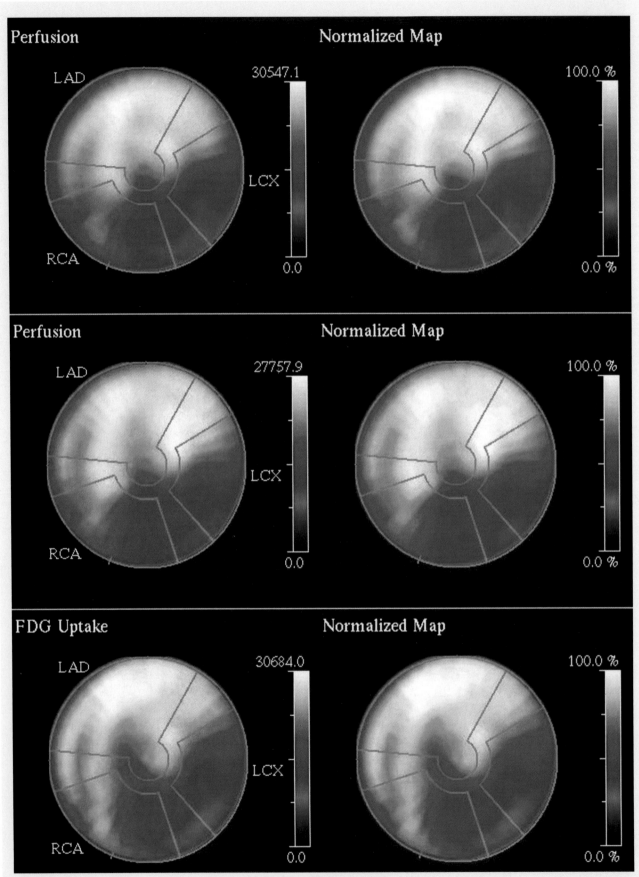

Figure 9.26

TABLE 9-1		
	Tl Redistribution	Sestamibi Nitrates
PPV	70%	79%
NPV	65%	74%

Data from Sciagrà RV, Bisi G, Santoro GM, et al. Comparison of baseline-nitrate technetium sestamibi with rest-redistribution thallium-201 tomography in detecting viable hibernating myocardium and predicting postrevascularization recovery. *J Am Coll Cardiol.* 1997;30:384–391.

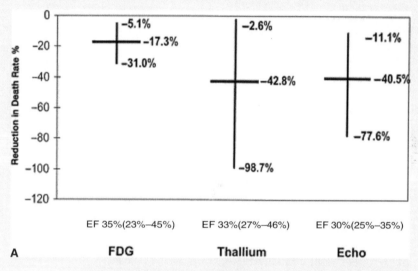

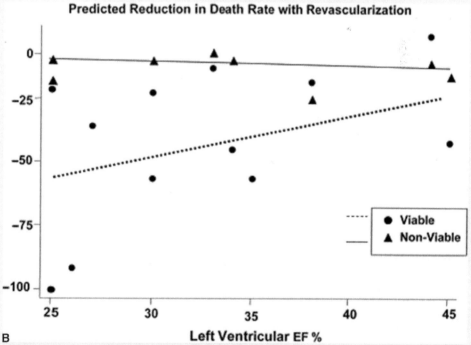

Figure 9.27 Reprinted from Allman KC, Shaw LJ, Hachamovitch R, et al. Myocardial viability testing and impact of revascularization on prognosis in patients with coronary artery disease and left ventricular dysfunction: a meta-analysis. *J Am Coll Cardiol.* 2002;39:1151–1158, with permission from Elsevier.

26. ANSWER: E. All of the statements are true.

27. ANSWER: A. Patients with diabetes have a higher calcium score and higher mortality than patients without diabetes. These observations were made by Raggi P, Shaw LJ, Berman DS, et al. Prognostic value of coronary artery calcium screening in subjects with and without diabetes. *J Am Coll Cardiol.* 2004;43(9):1663–1669.

28. ANSWER: A. Patients with and without diabetes and zero calcium score have very low and similar event rates at 5 years. No further risk stratification is needed. These observations were made by Raggi P, Shaw LJ, Berman DS, et al. Prognostic value of coronary artery calcium screening in subjects with and without diabetes. *J Am Coll Cardiol.* 2004;43(9):1663–1669.

29. ANSWER: B. Patients with diabetes and those with metabolic syndrome have a blunting of heart rate response to adenosine and regadenoson that is attributed to cardiac autonomic neuropathy. There is a direct relationship between the blood sugar level on the day of the stress test and the heart rate response both in diabetic patients and also in patients not known to be diabetic. Patients with blunted heart rate response to pharmacologic stress testing have a high mortality compared to patients with normal heart rate response.

REFERENCES:

Hage FG, Dean P, Bhatia V, et al. The prognostic value of the heart rate response to adenosine in relation to diabetes mellitus and chronic kidney disease. *Am Heart J.* 2011;162(2):356–362.

Hage FG, Dean P, Iqbal F, et al. A blunted heart rate response to regadenoson is an independent prognostic indicator in patients undergoing myocardial perfusion imaging. *J Nucl Cardiol.* 2011;18(6):1086–1094.

30. ANSWER: E. All of these findings have been reported in diabetic patients and cardiac autonomic dysfunction.

REFERENCE:

Hage FG, Iskandrian AE. Cardiovascular imaging in diabetes mellitus. *J Nucl Cardiol.* 2011;18(5):959–965.

31. ANSWER: A. CZT detectors were recently introduced. They tend to be more expensive than the traditional dual SPECT detectors. However, they use a multipinhole design and simultaneous multiview acquisition to improve the energy and spatial resolution. The ultimate result is reduction in dosimetry (radiation) and image acquisition time.

32. ANSWER: C. Calcium deposition in the coronary arteries is often a late phenomenon in the atherosclerotic process and a reflection of earlier soft plaque rupture and subsequent healing. It is a very specific indicator of atherosclerotic plaque burden. It is not very sensitive for the presence of plaques since it misses the soft noncalcified plaque. Calcium is often present in the absence of any symptoms.

33. ANSWER: C. MDCT of calcium scoring does not require contrast media and slice thickness of around 3 mm. It is generally recommended for patients with low-to-intermediate likelihood for CAD, and under these circumstances, effective radiation dose should follow the as low as reasonable achievable (ALARA) principles and be under 3 mSv.

REFERENCE:

Voros S, Rivera JJ, Berman DS, et al.; Society for Atherosclerosis Imaging and Prevention Tomographic Imaging and Prevention Councils; Society of Cardiovascular Computed Tomography. Guideline for minimizing radiation exposure during acquisition of coronary artery calcium scans with the use of multidetector computed tomography: a report by the Society for Atherosclerosis Imaging and Prevention Tomographic Imaging and Prevention Councils in collaboration with the Society of Cardiovascular Computed Tomography. *J Cardiovasc Comput Tomogr.* 2011;5(2):75–83.

34. ANSWER: D. CAC provides incremental value for favorable or unfavorable risk stratification, as compared to traditional risk factors like FRS. This concept has been validated even in ethnic minorities (MESA study). A zero calcium score predicts very low event rates irrespective of other risk factors.

REFERENCE:

Sarwar A, Shaw LJ, Shapiro MD, et al. Diagnostic and prognostic value of absence of coronary artery calcification. *JACC Cardiovasc Imaging.* 2009;2:675–688.

35. ANSWER: C. CAC > 1,000, predicts short-term events (1 year) exceeding 25% versus 7.5% seen in patients with very abnormal MPI SPECT. This is seen in symptomatic or asymptomatic patients.

REFERENCE:

Wayhs R, Zelinger A, Raggi P. High coronary artery calcium scores pose an extremely elevated risk for hard events. *J Am Coll Cardiol.* 2002;39(2):225–230.

36. ANSWER: A. These two modalities were found to be complementary in terms of risk prediction in multiple studies. Rozanski et al. found that patients with normal SPECT MPI have a low event rate irrespective of their calcium score. However, when patients have a high-risk MPI SPECT and a high CAC, the 10-year mortality is 42%, compared to around 30% when only one of the tests is abnormal.

REFERENCES:

Chang SM, Nabi F, Xu J, et al. The coronary artery calcium score and stress myocardial perfusion imaging provide independent and complementary prediction of cardiac risk. *J Am Coll Cardiol.* 2009;54(20):1872–1882.

Rozanski A, Gransar H, Wong ND, et al. Clinical outcomes after both coronary calcium scanning and exercise myocardial perfusion scintigraphy. *J Am Coll Cardiol.* 2007;49(12):1352–1361.

37. ANSWER: B. Asymptomatic patients undergoing PET MPI and CAC scoring who have a normal MPI and a CAC < 100 have no events as compared to patients with normal MPI and a CAC > 1,000 who have an event rate of >10%. Patients with normal MPI and CAC > 400 have an event rate 2.9 times higher than patients with normal MPI and CAC < 400.

REFERENCE:

Schenker MP, Dorbala S, Hong EC, et al. Interrelation of coronary calcification, myocardial ischemia, and outcomes in patients with intermediate likelihood of coronary artery disease: a combined positron emission tomography/computed tomography study. *Circulation.* 2008;117(13):1693–700.

38. ANSWER: C. A typical SPECT MPI exposes patients to 12 to 16 mSv of radiation versus 3.7 mSv for PET rubidium-82 and 2.3 mSv for PET NH_3.

REFERENCE:

Senthamizhchelvan S, Bravo PE, Esaias C, et al. Human biodistribution and radiation dosimetry of 82Rb. *J Nucl Med.* 2010;51(10):1592–1599.

39. ANSWER: E. All of the methods have been proposed to minimize radiation exposure when undergoing SPECT MPI testing.

40. ANSWER: D. The sensitivity of SPECT MPI is reduced when patients are on beta-blockers irrespective of the stress modality or the ability to reach target heart rate. Also, the size of the perfusion defect is often smaller or absent.

REFERENCES:

Hockings B, Saltissi S, Croft DN, et al. Effect of beta adrenergic blockade on thallium-201 myocardial perfusion imaging. *Br Heart J.* 1983;49(1):83–89.

Reyes E, Stirrup J, Roughton M, et al. Attenuation of adenosine-induced myocardial perfusion heterogeneity by atenolol and other cardioselective beta-adrenoceptor blockers: a crossover myocardial perfusion imaging study. *J Nucl Med.* 2010;51:1036–1043.

41. ANSWER: D. Caffeine, theophylline, and ʟ-arginine (a nitrate precursor) should be stopped prior to pharmacologic stress testing to prevent blunting of vasodilation and therefore underestimation of ischemia. Despite their impact on endothelial function, there are no current recommendations to stop statins prior to testing.

42. ANSWER: C. Adenosine is a potent vasodilator that also increases the heart rate at low dose by vagal inhibition. Adenosine has the potential to cause bradycardia at high dose, and it has no known direct inotropic effects.

43. ANSWER: A. Combination of exercise with pharmacologic stress testing can reduce the duration of side effects, decrease liver activity, and improve the sensitivity to detect ischemia, in addition to providing a window on the functional capacity of patients referred for risk stratification. However, by increasing the heart rate, exercise can lead to more artifacts in patients with LBBB.

REFERENCES:

Candell-Riera J, Santana-Boado C, Castell-Conesa J, et al. Simultaneous dipyridamole/maximal subjective exercise with 99mTc-MIBI SPECT: improved diagnostic yield in coronary artery disease. *J Am Coll Cardiol.* 1997;29(3):531–536.

Holly TA, Satran A, Bromet DS, et al. The impact of adjunctive adenosine infusion during exercise myocardial perfusion imaging: results of the Both Exercise and Adenosine Stress Test (BEAST) trial. *J Nucl Cardiol.* 2003;10(3):291–296.

Vitola JV, Brambatti JC, Caligaris F, et al. Exercise supplementation to dipyridamole prevents hypotension, improves electrocardiogram sensitivity, and increases heart-to-liver activity ratio on Tc-99m sestamibi imaging. *J Nucl Cardiol.* 2001;8(6):652–659.

44. ANSWER: D. The most common adverse events with adenosine use are second-degree AV block (4.1%), hypotension (1.8%), bradycardia (0.2%), and third-degree AV block (0.8%).

REFERENCE:

Cerqueira MD, Verani MS, Schwaiger M, et al. Safety profile of adenosine stress perfusion imaging: results from the Adenoscan Multicenter Trial Registry. *J Am Coll Cardiol.* 1994;23(2):384–389.

45. ANSWER: A. Chest pain occurs in 20% of patients undergoing dipyridamole pharmacologic stress testing. Other events are less common.

REFERENCE:

Ranhosky A, Kempthorne-Rawson J. The safety of intravenous dipyridamole thallium myocardial perfusion imaging. Intravenous Dipyridamole Thallium Imaging Study Group. *Circulation.* 1990;81(4):1205–1209.

46. ANSWER: A. The use of a ramp filter during filtered back projection reconstruction will result in decreased counts in the wall of the left ventricle closest to the hot area. Iterative reconstruction lessens this effect of a hot liver or loop of bowel. Resolution recovery, correction for the loss of resolution the further an object is from the detector, should not influence the counts in an area. Scatter correction, correction for the overrepresentation in counts due to misregistration of counts coming from a hot area close to the heart, will decrease the total counts in the inferior wall. Of the possible options, A is the most likely answer.

47. ANSWER: A. Scaling or normalization artifacts occur with greater frequency in low-count studies using fixed threshold filtering during reconstruction. Obese patients have greater attenuation resulting in lower counts, and this effect is greater when doing 1-day studies with split doses as opposed to 2-day studies when equal and higher doses are given. Females in general have greater anterior wall attenuation due to the presence of breast tissue, and this is most likely to result in normalization problems or the creation of hot spots.

48. ANSWER: C. If the patient has a narrow complex, most ICD systems will differentiate sinus tachycardia from slow VT, and most of these protocols should work fine. In this particular patient, the wide QRS complex has a greater potential to cause confusion. Of the four options, adenosine alone will cause the lowest increase in heart rate and is the least likely to cause misinterpretation by the ICD. All of the others cause an increase in heart rate that may potentially reach the relatively low rate threshold for VT recognition.

49. ANSWER: C. Metal devices in the heart have the potential to cause artifacts when using CT attenuation correction. Most of the current SPECT/CT and PET/CT systems have recognized this and correct for such artifacts. The greater the extent of metal present, the more likely there is to be an artifact. ICD systems have the greatest metal content and are thus most likely to result in artifacts when using CT attenuation correction.

50. ANSWER: A. Due to the half-life of 72 seconds, stress-only rubidium-82 results in the lowest radiation exposure in the listed protocol options. All of the other agents have longer half-lives and will expose the patient to higher levels regardless if done with stress-only or in a 1-day sequence.

51. ANSWER: C. All of these agents have the potential to delay conduction in the atrioventricular node (AVN), but in the literature, dipyridamole is the least likely to cause block. The two selective A2A agonists, regadenoson and binodenoson, have reported a low occurrence of first- and second-degree block, while the nonselective A2A agonist, adenosine, is the most likely to cause AVN block due to stimulation of the A1 receptors in the AVN. Dipyridamole is not associated with blocking the AVN node. This may be due in part to the fact that dipyridamole depletes intracellular levels of adenosine in order to allow accumulation of endogenous adenosine in the extracellular space. The combination of low intracellular and high extracellular adenosine does not cause as much block. With adenosine, there is an increase in both intra- and extracellular adenosine, and this combination has a strong inhibitory effect on the AVN.

52. ANSWER: B. Counts, scatter, and attenuation are generally uniform across the field of view. The center generally has the greatest uniformity of crystal and photomultiplier tubes. At the edges of the field, light leaks due to poor contact between the photomultiplier tubes and the crystal that are glued together are more common. Placing the heart at the extreme edge also increases the chance that on some views the heart will be out of the field. This is especially a problem on systems that have pressure-sensitive detectors that will reorient when they get too close to the patient's body.

53. ANSWER: A. BGO and LSO are used for PET imaging detector systems as the response rate of these materials is optimal for the 511 keV photons. For use with technetium-99m–radiolabeled materials in single photon emission computed tomography systems, NaI is the most commonly used due to wider availability and lower cost, but it has a less efficient response rate than the CZT systems.

54. ANSWER: C. The postulated mechanism for using any of the above is that they either increase intestinal motility or push the loops of bowel toward the pelvis when the patient is supine during acquisition and gravity causes layering. Solid food, water, and coffee given in adequate quantities have greater attenuation than carbonated beverages, such as soda, which releases gas. The mixture of liquid and gas causes less attenuation than liquids and solids.

55. ANSWER: B. New onset of atrial fibrillation with a rapid response needs to be medically diagnosed and managed before any type of stress testing is performed. This is based on patient safety and the lack of diagnostic accuracy as there is not a true baseline blood flow measurement. Since the patient is unaware of the arrhythmia, it is probable he was in atrial fibrillation at the time of the resting study, which is then not a true baseline measure of blood flow. It likely will be the same as the stress study even if there is coronary disease present. It is not appropriate to temporarily lower the heart rate or administer adenosine to cause further coronary vasodilation as these measures can potentially lower blood pressure.

56. ANSWER: C. This patient has atypical symptoms and with an underlying LBBB requires further evaluation. With the LBBB, exercise with nuclear imaging is not the best test due to low specificity associated with exercised-induced septal perfusion defects. In a young female patient, it is important to give as low a radiation dose as possible. A dual-isotope study with exercise gives the highest radiation exposure with the lowest diagnostic accuracy. A technetium-99m study gives a lower radiation dose but when used in combination with exercise will have lower accuracy. Nitrogen-13 ammonia PET will give the lowest radiation dose from the radionuclide techniques, but the use of exercise may still be a problem. Stress echocardiography can diagnose the presence or absence of CAD and provides no radiation. In this situation, it may also provide useful information on nonischemic heart disease, which is a concern in the presence of the LBBB.

57. ANSWER: C. Interpreting the study as is will not be diagnostic based on the large distance moved. Since it is not possible to correct for side-to-side or horizontal motion, this is not an option and speaking to the patient and explaining the need to reacquire the images is the best step to get accurate results. Although stress echocardiography is acquired over a short time period and in this patient should give accurate results, the patient has already received the radiation exposure and performed exercise stress, so the most efficient way to get the results is to maximize accuracy of the available data.

58. ANSWER: D. The residual background activity from the technetium-99m will interfere with a SPECT study, and in such a situation, delaying the SPECT MPI study 18 to 24 hours will give the most accurate results. Since surgery cannot be delayed that long and exclusion of ischemia is needed by the surgeons, an MPI study with the higher-energy 511 keV photons with PET will give the answer on the presence of CAD in the required time frame. Management in case of a positive study is complicated, but if the study is negative, the patient can be cleared for surgery.

59. ANSWER: A. Of these options, increasing the imaging time will increase counts the most and optimize accurate image interpretation. Prone imaging is useful for differentiating diaphragmatic attenuation from inferior infarction but does not improve count statistics in low-count studies. An ultrahigh-resolution collimator decreases the total counts. Administering 10 mCi in the resting state when blood flow in ischemic and normal areas is similar increases total counts but may lessen contrast for areas that were ischemic during stress.

60. ANSWER: A. Whole-body fluorine-18 FDG PET studies looking for primary tumors or metastases require overnight fasting to maximize tumor uptake of the tracer. Cardiac PET studies for viability attempt to drive glucose into myocytes, and blood glucose levels are routinely checked at baseline. If levels are too low, D50 can be administered, and if they are too high, insulin on a sliding scale is administered so that when fluorine-18 FDG is administered, it is not diluted out by the high endogenous glucose levels. After administration of fluorine-18 FDG, glucose levels are again checked and an attempt is made to drive glucose into cells. Thus, 12-hour fasting assures that glucose levels are not too elevated. Longer fasts are not necessary.

61. ANSWER: D. The large and small fields of view dual-headed systems do not allow optimal positioning of the camera head relative to the patient that permits the best septal view LAO. Since most are in a fixed 90-degree configuration and do not allow caudal tilt angulation, this limits the rotation. The single-headed large field of view extends too far toward the abdomen to allow angulation. The single-headed small field of view is generally not produced as acquisition times for single photon emission computed tomography are longer but for MUGA studies provides the best flexibility for angulation.

INDEX

Note: Page numbers in *italics* refer to figures, and those followed by 't' refer to tables.